INTERMITTENT FASTING

The complete beginner's and advanced guide for
quick weight loss
to burn fat, stay healthy, and gain energy with
alternate day fasting

Table of Contents

Introduction

The commitment to improving your wellness and losing weight is superb as you have managed to reach this point. Losing weight is not an easy feat to accomplish, however, your life will surely change in ways you could not even imagine if you can follow the guiding principles you have studied in this book and remain motivated. You are on the correct path to improving both your physical and mental health. You will feel great, be secure from many prevalent nutritional illnesses, have elevated power levels, better personal appreciation, as well as other changes in your system. Your life will be significantly enhanced.

We are all not the same, both internally and externally, so you should spend time to know the implications of a weight loss program and attempt it slowly at first. It is not recommended to immerse yourself in a weight loss program you don't understand as you may not be able to follow it for long. No, IF regiment works flawlessly for all, so when choosing one, change it accordingly to suit your needs. There is a large number of weight loss programs, but some may be too difficult to pursue or simply unsafe. The amount of activity and the number of activities you take part in your life should be another significant consideration when picking a fasting regiment. It operates better if you do it consistently on a set routine.

Closely monitor your experiences and generally try to understand yourself more. Begin to collect information, gain an understanding of your system, and derive conclusions to direct your future actions. You ought to give your system time, especially because adapting to your new program generally requires a few weeks. You'll experience ups and downs, but that happens in everything in life. You will find ways to get more "ups" by remaining open-minded and not being overwhelmed by the "downs." Focus on the performance of the method, not the result. IF is an excellent way to boost yourself psychologically, but you must be aware of how your system reacts to an IF program. This is because your body system determines what you eat, how long you spend eating, how long you exercise, how many calories you eat, etc. But it's not about eating whenever you feel like. It implies being keen on how nutrition and fasting affect it. Given all of these factors, your fasting program, and ultimately, your weight will be under control. So, once you regulate your nutrition and IF program, you will be fully in command of your weight reduction process.

Being in a hurry to lose fat will not help you achieve your goals faster. Many individuals are too eager to burn fat that they interchange one IF regiment with another because they think that they don't operate fast enough. You need to know that the reduction of weight is supposed to be slow so that you remain healthy.

To get maximum weight loss, you must try to do something. Start your day in the morning with eight glasses of water. It will assist you to begin your day being hydrated and put the tempo for water intake all day long. Try always to be active so that you can take your thoughts away from food. Fasting on a busy day will show that being occupied can make you void being hungry. Make sure you take coffee because it is a gentle suppressant of hunger. There is also some proof of hunger suppression with green tea. Homemade bone broth and black coffee can also be used to regulate hunger. Keep in mind that hunger comes and goes. Get a bottle of water or coffee and take it slowly when you begin to feel famished. Your starvation will be gone by the time you have completed it.

You shouldn't let individuals know that you are fasting. This is because most individuals will attempt and deter you because they do not know the advantages of fasting. It's better to have a small group of people who fast than to seek help from people who don't fast since they understand how vital fasting is. As previously mentioned, it'll be difficult to start these regiments, but you must never stop trying. You should take nutritious food even on days you aren't fasting. Intermittent fasting isn't an allowance for eating anything you want. Try to adhere to a low-carb and low sugar food intake during the days you are not fasting. Eating food high in good fats can also keep your system in a fat-burning state, and ultimately, make fasting easier. Avoid overeating after fasting. Eat the regular amount you would have, as though you'd never fasted.

Chapter 1 Benefits of intermittent fasting

When it comes to your body, then you always want to know what the importance will be and how it will affect you. There are many advantages of intermittent fasting, just like the many surveys and research that was conducted on animals in laboratories. It was found that when animals were given foods on their specific time, they stayed fit and healthy. Those animals which were left free to eat as much as they wanted any time started having diseases. This was then converted to a report, and it was finalized that time scheduled eating was a great benefit for health. Hence it was decided to implement on humans.

People who eat without a schedule appeared to have more issues, and most of all, they had obesity in them. People who followed intermittent fasting showed remarkable signs and changes. Through research, it was found that the benefits of intermittent fasting included:

- A proven weight loss without the hassle of going to the gym or exercising.

- A lot of health benefits reducing diseases risks even cancer risks
- Proven brain health and mental stability

1. Reduction of type 2 Diabetes

Some studies show that even type 2 diabetes is reduced from intermittent fasting. It can even benefit the patients that have increased the risk of diabetes by lowering their diabetes level. It provides stability in their blood flow and immune system and helps the digestive system stay healthy. This results in a healthier body.

2. Beneficial to heart

Researches made in laboratories showed that intermittent fasting helps the cardiovascular system. A report in 2016 was conducted and proved that intermittent fasting reduces all kinds of issues like blood pressure, triglycerides, cholesterol, and even heart rate in animals as well as humans.

3. Healthy Brain

Intermittent fasting shows that mental stability is possible, and it provides perfect brain health. Through this, a person stays fresh mentally; he does not feel extra burdened and stressed. Nor does his brain feels tired. A healthy and fresh brain is the achievement of many successes and solutions to many problems.

Your thoughts will be clear. You will stay in peace; you will have the ability to analyze things at a quicker pace. This is best for students as well as for people who have to workloads in offices. It helps them stay off the alert notice and helps them become successful. For students, it might be perfect in learning everything and stay at the top of the class (that is of course, only if you want to).

It gives you the ability to increase the power of your memory too! You can remember things at greater detail. You won't be disappointed by your own brain becoming a vault.

If you are someone who gets depressed a lot? Or, is your teen upset most of the time? Get yourself an intermittent fasting plan and stay healthy and fit. It relaxes your souls and body. It eases your mind. And it is perfect for hasty teens. There won't be any more depression affecting you. You might become just the perfect personality you always wanted to have. By just taking control over yourself, your brain, your soul, and your body.

4. Reduction of cancer

Studies showed that intermittent fasting reduced cancer even in animals. It later proved that humans were facing problems of cancer and the major reason for that was their diet plans. Hence following a planner will reduce the risks of cancer growing in your body.

The main reason for this is that obesity is the major reason for the growth of cancers most of the time. Through intermittent fasting, one loses weight and reduces the chance of obesity. This further reduces the chances of all issues or diseases that might grow in your body.

5. Boosting of biological processes

Biological processes play a massive role in our body's functionality. When you know how to boost your functions, your body interacts with matters at a greater rate. In order to be healthy, you need to know the answers to the questions, whether all hormones or chemicals in your body are balanced or not? If it is not like that then, there might be somethings imbalance in your body, which can cause any kind of illness or cellular degradation, which further leads to premature death! Hence, we need to take care of these questions and find solutions. The best solution is to perform intermittent fasting. This process will keep all your processes stable and in perfect order. It will also boost your biological systems, making you active in every activity that you want to perform or operate.

As it is said, people do not use their brains even up to 1%. The main reason for that is, they are stressed. Their entire system is stressed, not just their mind! This is the cause of eating at irregular times. Thus, if you set your schedule, you'll be able to control yourself rather than being controlled subconsciously.

When a person is under intermittent fasting and if he chooses to not eat for a longer time, then the body of that person goes under the autophagy process. The autophagy process is a process in which the old cells are cleared, and new cells take place. This process is only possible when a person stays without eating food for a certain period. It helps to ingest the components of the old cell and grow new ones. The new ones can only grow in the absence of old cells. When a person eats something, the glucose can create hindrances in the autophagy process hence try to drink only water or herbal tea during your fast.

Here are some important reasons showing you why intermittent fasting is important for you:

A study went on for 16 weeks, which was conducted on 283 people. Later it was found that people who ate breakfast, and people who didn't eat breakfast had no difference. Basically, it is considered a myth when people say breakfast is very essential, and if you don't eat it, you'll become weak or have diseases. The report concluded that people observed children performing better who had taken their breakfasts. Well, what about those who didn't eat their breakfasts? Some kids perform equally well without any problem. The reason is that it completely depends on the body of what it needs. If it can work even without breakfast or not. It is not essential, though.

There was another survey which denied everyone's assumption that eating more boosts your metabolism rate and burns fats. Well, this process is basically known as the thermic effect of food. It does not depend on how much you eat. It depends on how much calories you take in. For instance, if you are eating six times a day consisting of 500 calories, that's a lot excessive. But if you eat 3 meals consisting of 1000 calories, then it's the same deal. It will burn 300 calories in both ways. Hence it does not depend on the number of meals. It depends on your calorie intake.

People even believe that if they eat frequently, it will reduce their hunger. However, it is another myth, and it is completely wrong. Just like sleeping cycles, the more you sleep, the more your sleep will increase. The more you eat, the more your hunger will increase. It will not reduce; rather, it will make your body used to eat more without any hesitation. So, if you think that eating more will boost your metabolism rate, you are wrong. There's no difference. Studies showed that whether you eat three times or even 6 times a day, your metabolism rate depends on your body. Eating frequently will definitely not boost it.

One other common misbelief among people is, our body needs glucose for our brain to function with improvement. Our brain indeed needs glucose, but, that does not mean you eat carbs as much as you can to boost your brainpower. If your brain needs glucose, then your body will produce glucose itself for your brain. This process is known as gluconeogenesis. Even if you are starving for three days, your body can still produce the required glucose for itself. Hence you don't need to do your best in eating sweet stuff all the time. That doesn't mean not eating either. If you are on a long intermittent fasting process and feel dizzy, it is better to eat something light right away.

Some people even fuss over a myth known as protein distribution over meals. They believe that their body can only handle 30 grams per meal. Well, that is again incorrect. Protein intakes are not depended on a number of meals. It depends on how much protein you eat for your body to handle. And the metabolism rate definitely stays unaffected from protein intakes.

One other common disbelief that is shocking itself is, people, say that intermittent fasting will make you lose your muscle mass. Strictly speaking, these people do diet instead of intermittent fasting, and that is what reduces their muscle mass. Dieting is never healthy. Even bodybuilders are following the methods of intermittent fasting to help them maintain their muscle mass. So, it is clear that it will not eat your muscles away, but dieting surely will! A survey was conducted, and the conclusion which shocked people was that intermittent fasting would actually maintain your muscle mass. Hence this method is very popular among the community.

You might have even heard that intermittent fasting will not affect you only make your health go worse. The truth is it can not only improve body functionality; it has proven to increase a person's as well as animal's lifespans. It is basically the healthiest possible way to live by. Studies showed that this process could also increase your immunity and gene longevity. It has also proven to boost the health of BDNF (brain-derived neurotrophic factor), which is basically a hormone that protects against mental disorders.

Some people even protested that intermittent fasting makes you overeat due to extreme hunger. Well, you might indeed eat a bit more at the end of the day. That is because your body will be deprived of insulin levels and norepinephrine. Also, the levels of (HGH) human growth hormones become low. That is why a person normally eats more. But that doesn't make you fat. You actually lose weight. According to a survey, 3 to 8% and 4 to 7 % of people lost belly fat and weight in 2 to 24 weeks by intermittent fasting. People are more than happy with the results.

Don't just jump to conclusions when it's a matter of your health. It's better to consult some sources and do some research yourself. Your body can handle hunger. It's your mind that gets bothered. You only feel hungry when you know that you haven't eaten. This is relatable for people who are mostly busy with their work. They lose track of time to have meals, and they know that they don't feel hungry at all while they are working. When you try this process, don't forget to occupy your brain.

At the start, you will have some difficulties because you might have the habit of eating all the time. Hence, stay safe and stay healthy with a diet plan and treating your time as the most important gift. Do everything at the right time. As you all have heard the phrase "Excess of everything is bad and wrong." The same goes for the case of eating excessively. Always maintain yourself while eating. It was also a fact that people who eat by always keeping a portion of their tummy empty, they were always fit and safe from health problems. Intermittent fasting provides you with all these benefits and keeps you safe from all the health issues. You may never need to see a hospital again even (as some reviews of followers).

Chapter 2 Types of Intermittent Fasting

Intermittent fasting has different forms, and each can have a specific set of unique benefits. Each kind of intermittent fasting has variations in the post-meal relationship. The benefits and effectiveness of these different protocols may differ individually, and it is essential to determine which one is best for you. Factors that can influence the choice include health goals, daily schedule/routine and current health status.

The most common types of IF are alternate day fasting, time-restricted feeding, and modified fasting.

☐ Alternate Day Fasting

This approach involves alternating days without total calories (from food or drinks) with days of free feeding and eating whatever you want.

It has been shown that this plan helps with weight loss, improves cholesterol, and triglyceride (fat) levels in the blood and improves markers of inflammation in the blood.

The main disadvantage of this form of intermittent fasting is that it is the most difficult to stay due to the hunger reported on fasting days.

☐   Modified fasting - Diet 5: 2

Modified fasting is a protocol with days scheduled for fasting, but rest days allow some food intake. In general, it is allowed to consume 20 to 25% of regular calories on fasting days; Therefore, if you frequently consume 2000 calories on standard feeding days, you will be allowed 400-600 calories on fasting days. Part 5: 2 of this diet refers to the ratio of days without fasting to days of fasting. Therefore, on this diet, you would typically eat for 5 consecutive days, then fast or reduce your calories to 20-25% for 2 straight days.

This protocol is excellent for weight loss, body composition and can also benefit from the regulation of blood sugar, fats, and inflammation. Studies have shown that the 5: 2 protocol is effective for weight loss, improves/decreases markers of inflammation in the blood (3), and shows signs of developing insulin resistance. In animal studies, this 5: 2 modified diet resulted in a decrease in fat, a reduction of hunger hormones (leptin) and an increase in protein levels responsible for improving fat burning and regulating sugar in blood (adiponectin)

The modified 5: 2 protocol is easy to follow and has a small number of adverse side effects that include hunger, reduced energy, and some irritability at the beginning of the program. Contrary to this, however, studies have also seen improvements such as reduced blood pressure, less anger, less fatigue, self-confidence, and a more positive mood.

☐   Time-restricted feeding

If you know someone who said you are intermittent fasting, this is probably a form of limited-time feeding. This is a type of intermittent fasting that is used daily and involves the consumption of calories only for a small portion of the day and fasting for the rest.

Daily fasting intervals with limited time can vary between 12-20 hours, and the most common method is 16/8 (fasting for 16 hours, calorie consumption by 8). For this protocol, the time of day is not essential, as long as you fast for a consecutive period and eat only for the allowed time. For example, on a limited feeding schedule of 16/8, a person can eat the first meal at 7:00 and the last meal at 15:00 (fasting from 15:00 to 7:00), while another person can eat the first meal at 1 pm and the last meal at 9 pm. (fast from 9 PM to 1 PM). This protocol is designed to be performed every day for long periods and is very flexible as long as it remains in the fast / food window.

Feeding time is one of the most natural methods of intermittent fasting to follow. Using this in conjunction with your daily work and sleep schedule can help you achieve optimal metabolic function. Limited time feeding is an excellent program for weight loss and body composition improvement, as well as some other general health benefits. The few human studies that have been conducted have noted significant weight reductions, blood glucose reductions and increases in cholesterol, with no changes in perceived tension, depression, anger, fatigue or confusion. Some other preliminary results from animal studies have shown a time-limited diet to protect against obesity, high insulin levels, fatty liver disease, and inflammation.

The easy application and promising results of limited-time nutrition can make this an excellent option for weight loss and prevention/management of chronic diseases.

In addition to the above, there are several other types of intermittent work, such as One Meal per Day (OMAD) and various kinds of extended employment.

For our challenge, I recommend a fast diet 5: 2. It turns out to be the most popular method among celebrities.

The fast 5: 2 diet plan that encourages followers to eat many foods with whole grain and nutritious grains, both fasting and feasting. Not only is it a healthier alternative to some popular fasting plans, but it is also much easier (and more enjoyable) to follow than some of the most extreme fasting diets.

Weight loss and body fat are more than temporary good looks; It's about feeling good, learning how to eat healthily and sustainably, and improving your overall health and quality of life. This is the mission of the 5: 2 fast diet.

Chapter 3 The Three Magic Keys

Our health doesn't just involve your weight or a number on the scale. You should have a healthy mind, body, and soul. You need to keep a clear head to be able to focus on what's important and solve your biggest issues. A healthy body carries you throughout your life. Your soul is your passion, motivation, and inspiration. These make up your overall health, and there are three magic keys to unlocking this potential. By combining these three essential parts, you will be able to increase and optimize the speed of autophagy. These three magic keys which could take you beyond places you ever imagined are the process of fasting, exercise, and a balanced and healthy diet.

Fasting

The best way that you will be able to induce autophagy within your body is through the use of fasting. This seems to be a popular trend among many health nuts in today's world, but it is much more than just a fad. Fasting is something that humans have been doing for centuries, yet it is emerging now as a cure-all rather than something associated with religion. In order to help kickstart your body's natural process of eating itself, fasting can give you the boost you need to see extra weight loss with little effort in other areas of your health.

When you think of dieting, many people imagine that they have to starve themselves. Fasting is much different than just starvation. It is a planned attempt at making sure that you are limiting the windows that you are eating. When there are individuals who starve themselves because of eating disorders like anorexia, this is associated with a mental urge in order to reduce deeper feelings of anxiety and depression. It is an irrational and more compulsive action. Fasting is planned out. You aren't depriving your body of anything for too long. You are picking out specific windows when you will want to reduce what you are eating and other times when you allow yourself to eat a healthy and balanced diet.

Many individuals want to lose weight for aesthetic purposes, but it is important that you are focusing on reducing your weight in order to better enable yourself to prevent many health conditions that you might experience as you get older.

Intermittent fasting isn't really focused on dieting in the same context of limiting what foods you do or don't eat.

The foods that you decide to consume will be entirely up to you. Some individuals do just fine eating the things they already do but pairing it with a more limited diet such as one that is low-calorie has been known to help individuals lose an even higher amount of weight quicker. It's not that fasting makes no difference in what you can and can't eat. It is simply a way to work with your body to help induce more of those moments where you limit what you're eating.

This can sound very scary to some people. The periods of fasting with intermittent fasting aren't usually more than 24 hours. This isn't 24-hour awake either, this is a time period where you might be able to sleep for portions of it in order to ease the challenge of sometimes having to skip food. Intermittent fasting isn't something that will require you to starve yourself for days at a time. Your body already goes through a natural period where it is experiencing limited calories when you are sleeping. Those breaks in between lunch and dinner are times like this as well. We have all skipped a meal before too just because it was easier than having to go out and buy food. Intermittent fasting (IF) is never going to be more than this.

When you are fasting, you are also allowed to drink as much coffee, tea, and water with lemon as you want. Some individuals will even eat some zero-calorie snacks and drink things like bone broth. During these periods you can also make sure that you are doing hobbies to distract you, so before you often realize you will already be able to induce a healthy period of fasting.

Fasting is also something that can help us when we are sick. It might be our body's way of fighting off infection. There are even animals who have been known to naturally fast in order to help them overcome certain illnesses. Fasting can help you regulate your blood sugar and make sure that you are controlling your insulin levels. By doing this alone you might be able to regulate your weight. If your family is often at high risk of cancer, or maybe has a history of health conditions, then this might be something that you consider as well in order to keep your health in check and aid in the prevention of various kinds of diseases.

This is an entirely natural process. Though there is emerging science around it and of course there are some risks, it is still something that we have been doing for as long as we have been recording history. When paired with other autophagy inducing diets, such as a ketogenic diet, you might be able to lose a large amount of weight and dramatically decrease your chances of having any health conditions in the near future.

Unfortunately, long periods of fasting are the only way to really induce autophagy at the moment, and things like a healthy diet and exercise will just increase that. Your body will still be going through periods of natural autophagy, but you will not be able to induce it if you aren't restricting your caloric intake at all. Though we all go through these types of process in our life, it's important to remember that we are still all different individuals. Some people will be able to start fasting for one week and see results at the very end of the week. Other individuals will have a little bit more trouble, finding that they have to experiment with different kinds of methods over the period of a month or longer in order to ever find the results that they want. Don't be discouraged by anything that you might read about someone else's experiences. We are going to provide you with the most popular and most effective methods of intermittent fasting so that you can find the results that you have been desiring. It is up to you to determine what works best for you based on your lifestyle and the things that will come most naturally to you. The more educated you are on all of this, the easier it will be to determine what is right and wrong.

Exercise

Exercise is another point of importance in this health journey for you. If you are not conscious of the way that this diet might be able to affect your health paired with exercise, then you are going to be missing out on a third of the benefit of your fasting abilities. Exercise is not easy for everyone. It might be something that immediately triggers you or makes you fearful that you are going to have to struggle with a certain part of your life. Some of us have gone through traumatic experiences that have made exercise a very difficult part of our lives. We might struggle to find the courage to make it to the gym or even go for a walk outside without having extreme fear and anxiety over this.

However, exercise is absolutely something that you need to start including in your life. It is only going to make your health more challenging to deal with later on if you don't start to move now. The first thing that you will have to do in order to include a healthy exercise regimen in your life is to stop thinking of exercise as something that has to be a competition. Maybe you have experienced things in your past that made it seem as though you were constantly being put up against someone else in a competitive way but remember that it doesn't have to be like this anymore. You are a strong person capable of anything and overcoming your exercise fears is certainly one of those.

It's also essential that we remember that exercise is a mental thing that you have to push past. Once you start to exercise, it becomes even easier to do it more and more. The more you implement methods of movement, the easier that each new thing will be to complete. The hardest part is getting started. It's very challenging to get up off the couch when all you want to do is sit around and relax! This will certainly be a challenge for anyone that is looking to start off with a newer and healthier lifestyle. Once you get on that treadmill or start going for walks every day, you realize that it's so easy to get through it. Just thirty minutes a day running can be better than doing nothing at all throughout the rest of your week. We procrastinate going to the gym for just thirty minutes for weeks at a time. All of those moments spent agonizing over not wanting to go could instead be just seconds that we actually do go and get the work done. It is a mental thing that we have to start to learn how to get over.

Of course, this is all easier said than done. Many individuals struggle with anxiety and depression, as well as other mental illnesses, that could be the reason that it's so much harder to keep going forward. Exercise can actually decrease some of the side effects of this, along with many other health benefits, so it's essential that we still consider this as an option.

Another health benefit of exercise is that it will build your overall endurance and aerobic power. When you can do this, your body will be able to function optimally. You can endure longer periods of time for other types of work. If you are fasting, then it can be easier to continue on if you are someone that regularly exercises because you have that mental endurance to keep going forward. Exercise makes it easier to do simple aerobic things as well, such as walk up a flight of stairs, or walk a short distance rather than wasting time and gas driving there. As we get older, our endurance only becomes weaker, so it's crucial that we start to build this now.

Your blood pressure is often disregarded until we get older. It's crucial that we start to manage our blood pressure now in order to prevent chronic hypertension, which is one of the biggest reasons that many individuals will wind up with heart disease. Your blood pressure also puts a toll on your overall stress levels, so the better you can enable yourself to manage and reduce your stress, the happier your life will be.

Overall, it is essential that we are taking care of our immune system. This is like our body's armor against many different illnesses, infections, and diseases. When you aren't exercising, you aren't helping your immune system to function optimally. Aging can also be slowed down when you are able to manage your body's immune system.

Fasting and autophagy will help to use your body's fat for an energy source. This is great for helping you to lose weight. However, when you exercise, you are also making your body need more energy. When more energy is needed, more fat will be taken to provide that. At the same time, exercise can turn your fat cells into muscle cells, giving you an even healthier body. When your physical body is healthy, this will make it even easier for the rest of your organs to function. You will breathe better, have a higher energy level, and this can make you even happier mentally. Not only will having all of these aspects in your life make it easier to be happier, but exercise increases positive mental health as well.

When you exercise, you start to release endorphins. These can help provide positive neurotransmitters to your brain and make up for any drop-in serotonin levels that you might be experiencing. It can also provide a distraction and a way for your mind to have something else to focus on rather than the things that might be stressing you out. You will be able to keep your mind active, lowering your chances of having a poor memory or low intelligence.

Don't be afraid of exercise! It is one of the most important parts of living a healthy lifestyle. When we help you build your healthy lifestyle plan, we will discuss what types of exercises and which regimens you might choose based on what is best for you!

Low-Calorie Diet

Choosing a low-calorie diet is going to be one of the best options for you to optimize your health. You will want to ensure that you are enabling yourself to have all the resources needed in order to live your best life. When you deprive your body of having a fighting chance, you are only setting yourself up for failure. In order to understand why it is such a good option to pick a low-calorie diet, we first have to really understand what a calorie is! The most important thing to know is that there are no two calories that are created equal. They are a unit of measurement, but what is measured will apply differently to various types of food.

A calorie isn't something that the food has in it, like sodium or carbohydrates. A calorie represents what energy it takes to process this food. A calorie is essentially an amount of heat energy, and it is important that you start to think of it in this way. There are things labeled to us as having only "100 calories," but why does that matter? We see a low number and think that this means that it's healthy, but it likely doesn't have anything else beneficial in it to us. It is better to eat something that is 500 calories with protein, healthy carbs, and so on, rather than something that is 100 calories with just sugar and fat that makes it taste good.

When the calories are decided within food, the carbohydrate, fat, and protein content is all determined in order to discover what this heat energy means. When you are picking out healthy foods, you can almost ignore the calories and instead focus on the fat, protein, and carbohydrate content. Your fats should always be far less than your protein and carbs, and they should all help to balance each other out. As your body processes different foods, some of that is going to be used for different parts of your body and through this complex process of breaking down, more energy might be used up, meaning having a lower calorie count didn't matter in the beginning anyway!

One example of why it is important to remember this distinction is through foods that have a high level of glucose versus a high level of fructose. They both have the same calories per amount, but glucose is used by your entire body, whereas fructose is really only broken down by your liver. Foods with fructose versus glucose are going to be not as great of an option, but they have the same calorie count. When picking between two foods, don't assume that just because they have the same calories that they are going to provide you with the same health benefits.

What is also important to remember about low-calorie foods is that you also need to ensure that you are picking things that are filling. You might grab a bag of candy because it only has 100 calories. However, it would likely do you better to eat some veggies with hummus, even though this might be 200 calories per serving. This is because it will provide your body with more energy to breakdown that food you are eating, and any food that you have already eaten. In addition to this, it will also make sure that you stay fuller longer. Later on, in the day, you might be tempted to overeat if you only had a few calories, whereas if you eat filling food, you can more easily fight through cravings that might break your diet.

If you are going to be exercising and fasting, then you are going to need to eat all the filling low-calorie foods that you can get your hands on. Even though, we know that not all calories are created equal, it's still crucial that you are picking a low-calorie diet because this is going to give you a good basis of health foods that will aid in your weight loss. The key thing to remember is to not fall for things that are labeled by their caloric intake. Instead, look for things that promote having fewer carbs or no added sugar. Even the top candy bars will have their number of calories somewhat large in order to make you think that it is healthy. Low calorie does not equal health. Low calorie but high in vitamins and minerals, healthy carbs, less sugar, and less fat is going to be the best option for you overall. When comparing two things that are 100 calories per serving, look next at the protein that they provide. Higher protein will always be a better option. Pick the one with less fat and less sugar as well. Don't be too afraid of carbohydrates, unless you are trying a ketogenic or carb-restricted diet, of course. If it has high carbs, check the sugar count as well. If it has a lower sugar count, then this indicates it's going to have a better amount of healthy carbohydrates.

Don't give yourself 0-calorie food all the time either. It can be tempting because many people will think that this is the way to a healthier body and excess weight loss. Your body is still going to need energy in order to lose weight. You have to provide energy for your metabolism to stay active. If you deprive your body all the time and don't give it anything good, then it will end up hurting you in the end. You might go into starvation mode and your metabolism could actually slow. During times when you eat, choose low-calorie, but not no-calorie. Your body will want to have plenty of energy so it can stay burning fat all throughout your fasting and your eating periods. Throughout the book, we are going to provide more healthy options for foods that you can start to include in your diet.

Chapter 4 What Should I Expect When I Get Started With Fasting?

Once you have gotten started with fasting, you may be nervous about what to expect. Most of us have rarely ever missed a meal unless we were sick, and we have spent most of our lives being told that fasting is very bad for our health.

For the first few fasts that you undertake, the situation may be difficult. If you can get through the first two or three, then things get easier, but be ready for a rough couple of days as you start to adjust. The hunger that bothers you, in the beginning, will start to dissipate a bit and can be quelled with the help of a drink of water. You may also deal with a few other issues, such as headaches and heartburn like we talked about before, but these often disappear after a few fasts.

Some people are going to experience more issues with their fast compared to others. No one is quite sure why some people have bigger problems, but it may have to do with the diet that you had before you began fasting. One cause of fasting being more difficult for some compared to others is a phenomenon that is known as metabolic inflexibility. This is when the body has become so used to that constant supply of carbs and sugar from food that it is out of practice, turning to our fat stores for energy, and the side effects can hit you hard. However, the body is very adaptive, and after just a few fasts, it will learn how to access those fat stores to keep you energized, and the side effects are going to fade.

There are a few different problems that a beginner faster may experience. Some of these include:

- Intense hunger: These hunger pains will come and go through the day. These pains are like waves, rather than something that just builds up, so you just need to find ways to distract yourself to make it easier.

- Headaches: These are common when you first start. Take some painkillers to help and drink plenty of fluids.

- Lightheadedness: Some people report feeling a bit lightheaded and spaced out when they go on a fast. When you get to your eating window, eat something a little bit salty.

- Feeling tired: This is going to happen because the body hasn't had time to learn how to access the stores of fat that you have as fuel. A salty drink can help with this.

- Lots of irritability: This can be a big problem when you are near the end of your fast. Planning out the meals that you are going to eat ahead of time can really help. Be aware that your temper may be short, learn how to stay calm or stay away from other people.

- Insomnia: Some people have trouble falling asleep when they go on their first few fasts.

The good news is that most of these are going to fade away within a week or less. Having a good meal plan when you first get started on your intermittent fast and sticking with it, can make a big difference in how well you feel and how successful the fast is. When meal planning, add in lots of nutrients and consider putting one of your bigger meals as the first one to help the body get enough food after going on the fast.

There are also a few things that you can do to reduce the side effects of an intermittent fast and help you be better prepared for this kind of eating plan. First, take it easy for the first few weeks. If you have a big project that is going to occur at work or another stressful situation at hand, then hold off getting started with intermittent fasting.

These situations are going to make you crave food all the time and can already give you headaches and irritability. Adding the intermittent fast on top of that will just make things worse. Consider taking a few days off work if you can or just pick a time that is less stressful and demanding on you to help you get the best results!

Meal planning is another option that you can choose. After you get done with a fast, especially during the first few times, you are going to be really hungry. The body is not used to going such a long time without eating, and as soon as you let it have something, it will want to gobble down as much as it can get ahold of. If you don't have a plan in place, you are going to eat everything in the kitchen and take on way too many calories in the process.

With a good meal plan, you can avoid this issue. You can set up your meals ahead of time, especially for those eating periods right after your fast is ending. That way, when the fast is done, you can just grab the prepared meal and enjoy it, knowing that the meal has all the good nutrients that your body needs and will fill you up.

One thing to remember about meal planning with intermittent fasting is to consider making the first meal after a fast a little bit bigger. Many of us save supper as our biggest meal, but when you are done with a fast, the body is hungry and has been going for a long time without anything to eat. You can certainly provide yourself with a tiny meal after the fast, but you will end up hungry and dissatisfied. A better option is to add a bit more to that first meal to help provide the body with nutrients and to make it feel better. This can make the fast more enjoyable and will ensure you don't go and raid the fridge simply because you are still hungry after your fast.

Chapter 5 Eating On An Intermittent Fast

Eating on the intermittent fast can be as simple or as complicated as you choose to make it. Some people will continue with their healthy eating ahead of time, and others will add another type of diet to this one to see results. For example, the ketogenic diet can work well with this option because it helps to limit your carbs to reduce hunger and burn fat more quickly. However, it's not essential for you to go on any one specific diet plan to see results when on an intermittent fast.

The first thing to keep in mind is that it is not recommended that you eat unhealthy food when you are on this kind of diet plan. It is good to cut down your window of eating during the day to eight hours or less (or to do one of the other options for intermittent fasting), but, if you spend that time eating desserts, fast food, and other unhealthy foods, you will run into problems.

First, you will not be able to lose weight when you eat this way. Fast foods and other unhealthy choices come with many calories and sugar per serving, and it's likely that you are taking in more than one serving at a time. So, even though your window for eating is smaller, you can still take in too many calories which will stop all your weight loss progress. Even though intermittent fasting is not about the calorie intake, you still need to be cautious about eating too many calories because it's an aspect that can ultimately affect the effectiveness of intermittent fasting.

You will also notice that when you eat these unhealthy foods, even while on an intermittent fast, that you will not improve your health. Your health relies on good food that is high in nutrients to keep you strong. If you're simply fasting while still eating unhealthy food, this will likely cause just as many problems as you encountered before you started fasting.

When you eat these bad foods, you will find that you are hungry more often and you will struggle with getting through your fasting periods. This is because many processed and fast foods contain chemicals and preservatives that are designed to make you hungry more often. If you want to see results and get through your fast without feeling hungry, then it is time to eat foods that are better for you.

Now, this doesn't mean that you can't eat sweets or junk food occasionally. In fact, the intermittent fast doesn't have set rules for exactly what you can eat; it simply sets the times that you are allowed to eat. Eating a small cheat meal is fine if you have it during your eating windows and only do it on occasion. It may be hard sometimes but eating healthier will give you better results.

The trick to making the intermittent fast work for you is to eat a healthy diet. The more nutrients you can fit into your diet plan, the better you will end up doing with this fast.

The first thing that you need to consider is eating plenty of fruits and vegetables. Fresh produce is best because it provides lots of essential nutrients that your body needs to stay healthy. Consider filing your plate with fruits and vegetables each meal so that you are getting the nutrients that you need. Eating a wide variety of produce is also important to ensure that you are getting what your body needs without adding in too many calories.

Next, you should go with some good sources of protein. You should consider going with options like lean ground beef, turkey, and chicken. Having some bacon and other fatty meats on occasion is fine, just don't overdo it. Additionally, eating a lot of fish will help you to get the healthy fatty acids that the body needs to function properly.

Healthy sources of dairy also help you to stay lean while giving your body the calcium it needs. You can have some options such as milk, yogurt (be careful of the kinds that have fruit and other things added because these usually include a high amount of sugar), sour cream, cheese, etc., and be sure to monitor the salts and sugars that are not healthy for the body.

You can also have carbs on this diet. Recently, carbs have gotten a bit of a bad reputation because so many diet plans recommend that you avoid them, but the important thing here is to eat the carbs that are healthy for you. White bread and pasta are basically sugar in disguise and should be avoided, but choosing whole grain and whole wheat options when it comes to your carbs will ensure that you get all the nutrition that you need without all the "bad" carbs.

Having a well-balanced diet will be the key to ensuring that you feel good when you are on an intermittent fast. You will be able to mix up the meals that you choose so that you get the best results when you go on this kind of a fast.

You are also allowed to have a snack and treats as long as you are careful with how often this happens. If you are eating junk, you will be disappointed when you go to the scale and see that you are not losing weight.

Using the Ketogenic Diet with Intermittent Fasting

Lots of people decide to go on a ketogenic diet while doing an intermittent fast to help stay healthy. The ketogenic diet is a high fat, moderate protein, and low carb diet that will help you to burn fat quickly while reducing your dependence on carbs. There is a lot to love with this diet plan, and when it is combined with the intermittent fasting, you are sure to get some great results in no time.

It's possible to use both of these diet plans together. Intermittent fasting is focused on the times of day when you will eat, while the ketogenic diet on what to eat during those time periods. For those who would like to balance their blood sugar level and lose weight more efficiently, combining these two diet plans together can be a great option.

With intermittent fasting, you are limiting the hours that you eat. Instead of spreading your meals and your snacks throughout the day, you will limit it to just a few hours. Many people choose to only eat between 10am and 6pm and fit their macronutrients into that time. Others, however, will take two or three days during the week where they are not allowed to eat and fit their nutrients into the other days of the week.

The point is that you are limiting the amount of time that you eat, thereby forcing yourself to think more about the foods you consume. You also get the benefit of more fat burning and weight loss, when you do intermittent fasting.

This means that you will still stick with high fat, moderate protein, and low carb diet plan even while intermittent fasting. You will just need to be more careful about the times you eat those macronutrients, but otherwise, you can follow the ketogenic diet exactly the same.

If you want to get some of the benefits of intermittent fasting or want to increase your weight loss, then adding this diet in with the ketogenic diet can be effective. You can experiment with the different types of intermittent fasting options that are available to see which one fits into your schedule the best or works the best for you. Of course, if you find the ketogenic diet is effective or intermittent fasting is too difficult, you can always just stick with the ketogenic diet and not fast and still see good results.

It is important to remember that you don't have to follow the ketogenic diet if you don't want to while on an intermittent fast. Many people do choose other healthy diets over the ketogenic diet, but many still choose to go with the ketogenic diet along with intermittent fasting because it is easy to follow and will allow them to lose even more fat.

Eating on the intermittent fast does not need to be too difficult. You can pick out the foods that you want to eat, although it is important to go with foods that are fresh and whole and will fill you up and help with the fat burning process to help you to see the weight loss that you are looking for.

Chapter 6 Food Choices

When you eat, food is broken down into molecules that flow through the bloodstream into your cells and organs. Carbohydrates, in particular, are broken down into a sugar which the body uses for energy, if your cells don't use, or need all of the energy supplied it gets stored in your fat cells to be used later on, and if all of that energy isn't used it stays in your body as that undesired fat you may wish to shed. This sugar energy needs insulin to enter your cells and do its work, so when you eat anything, not just carbs, your body produces insulin in order to process the energy you have provided. When you fast, and even when you don't snack between meals, the levels of insulin in your body become low enough for long enough that your body is triggered to source the energy from what has been stored in your fat cells, essentially burning fat.

To better understand how fasting can affect your metabolism, you first must understand the basic building blocks within your food and how they are processed in the body. The main nutrients needed in the greatest abundance are carbohydrates, proteins, and fats, and these are collectively known as macronutrients.

Nutrients needed in smaller doses that help with human development are the vitamins and minerals found in all foods, and these are collectively known as micronutrients. These come to us in two forms, one is needed daily, and the other can be stored in the body for use when needed. The majority of strategic nutrition plans focus on macronutrients as they are the literal building blocks of our DNA, they are required in a high volume, and they have the most immediate impact on metabolism in the form of insulin, hormones and stored energy sources.

Carbohydrates

If you've read anything about losing weight or healthy eating you've probably heard about a low-carb diet, which is simply restricting the number of carbohydrates (AKA carbs) that you eat, but carbs are an essential building block, and they exist in almost every food you will ingest. When you think "Carbs" you probably think bread, pasta or rice, but carbs exist in vegetables, fruits, and most beans. So how do you have a low carb diet when carbs are in everything?

Carbohydrates, to your metabolism, are basically starch and sugar, and when broken down, a carb is simply a form of energy called glucose. The important factor to consider is what level of energy do you want to provide your body. Carbs like bread, pasta, and rice get broken down and hit your metabolism with a spike of this form of energy which has a cascading effect on your hormones that regulate the rest of your body's systems. Major spikes and drops in hormones such as insulin and glucagon can have a lasting effect on your overall health and may lead to larger health problems if not managed properly over long periods of time.

The main goal is to maintain a controlled supply of glucose in the blood (aka blood sugar) and avoid any unnecessary spikes and shortages. By getting the majority of your carbohydrates from fruits, vegetables, and beans, you can reduce the spikes created from large volumes of pasta, bread, and other starchy grains. This isn't to say you should enjoy those foods, but they need to be in moderation and come second to the carbs available through other sources. Carbohydrates are one of the main sources of fuel for brain functions, so the body has become very efficient at storing the glucose found in carbs, and when you fast you remove the easily accessible fuel source and force your body to rely on the energy stored, creating a need to release, rebuild and cleanse out the systems that operate these functions.

There are so-called 'good carbs' which can provide the fuel needed without creating major glucose spikes and should be enjoyed in moderation and then there are 'bad carbs' which should be avoided or limited to a once-in-a-while indulgence

"Good carbs" include:

Vegetables: potatoes and beets, corn

Fruits: bananas, blueberries, oranges, grapefruits, apples

Grains: quinoa, buckwheat, oats, sprouted whole wheat

Beans: chickpeas, kidney beans, lentils "Bad carbs"

include:

Sugars: baked goods, soda, fruit juices

Processed: white bread, pasta, rice, chips crackers, etc.

Proteins

In any fitness magazine, you will likely come across the discussion of how to get enough protein, especially if the goal is to grow muscles - everyone wants to "get those gains." But the truth is we don't necessarily need more protein, you need the best proteins at the right time, and the sources of proteins can be surprising, as in, not only from meat.

Protein is the actual building block for rebuilding and repairing our DNA through the use of the 'essential amino acids' which are only available to humans through the nutrients they ingest, your body needs them to survive and cannot produce them on its own so relies on the nutrients provided by the food you consume to carry out the processes needed to generate energy and create new proteins which can then be used to grow and repair the body.

Your metabolism will take the whole protein sources you provide and break them down into increasingly smaller and more functional amino acids which are then carried in the bloodstream to your cells and reassembled as needed though protein synthesis within the cell structure. With a balanced diet, you will receive the required amino acids, and the body can function efficiently; however, if you are not consuming enough calories, your body may turn to other sources, such as your own muscle tissue as a source of these amino acids. This is not a concern with fasting, though, as the body is trained to store nutrients as energy and access the sources as needed and can absorb proteins quickly once consumed. If too much protein is consumed the body stores the amino acids as fat, so during a fasting window, this is the first place the body looks for fuel and not in the muscle tissues. During the eating window consuming the level of proteins needed for your specific body and goals and then letting the body access those stores during the fasting window you create a system in which the body has everything it needs and no more, and allows your fat cells to act as a warehouse for energy that is depleted on a regular basis instead becoming overloaded.

Healthy sources of protein include:

Soy: tofu, tempeh edamame

Pulses: lentils, peas, kidney beans, chickpeas

Seeds: pumpkin, flax, chia, sunflower

Animal products: seafood, poultry, eggs, some dairy (minimally processed)

Fats

Dietary fats have gotten a bad reputation in the world of fad diets; even the word "fat" gets some people nervous, how can a fat help with weight loss? As with all nutrients, there are 'good fats' and so-called 'bad fats,' and the body needs healthy fats to work its magic. The body uses the nutrients in dietary fats for brain development, heart functions, and the absorption of some key vitamins and a steady supply of healthy fats can produce softer, younger-looking skin and shiny healthy-looking hair.

Healthy dietary fats are a source of energy for the body and are where the body likes to store the excess energy from the other macronutrients consumed. The liver produces and stores the majority of this energy, and when you are in a fasting window, this is where the body turns for the energy needed to function. Fats are a concentrated energy source, meaning they have a high ratio of energy per calorie, this means you don't need to consume a lot of dietary fat to receive a huge dose of nutritional energy. This concentrated energy also provides an increased feeling of satiety, meaning they fill you up more than carb or protein would, so including some healthy fats into each meal will mean you can eat less and feel fuller and for a longer period of time. This will help you throughout your fasting window with cravings and the urge to eat something. By having a good portion of dietary fat with the first meal of your eating window you can ensure you provide the body with a strong source of fuel to absorb and utilize throughout the rest of your day.

Healthy dietary fats include:

Coconut products: oil, milk, amino, flakes

Avocado & Olives: whole or as an oil (drizzled on salads, not for high heat cooking)

Nuts: whole or in a nut butter

Seeds: chia, pumpkin, fax

Fish: salmon, mackerel, cod liver oil

Supplements: Omega 3 and Omega 6 daily supplements

Intermittent fasting is a strategic method of nutrient intake with the purpose of providing the body with the opportunity to utilize the stored energy provided. By selectively putting the body under the mild stress of a 'starvation' mode it allows your body to efficiently use up all the energy provided instead of storing the excess energy in the form of undesired fat. Through a balanced diet of whole foods, preferably organic when possible and limiting the so-called 'bad foods' you give your body everything it needs to function at its best.

Chapter 7 What Is Allowed When I Am Fasting?

Many people wonder what they are allowed to eat during their fasted state. They understand that they need to avoid drinks with calories and food and snacks during this time. However, what about some of the items that may not be considered as food, such as gum, breath mints, and even medications? These can provide a type of gray area when it comes to intermittent fasting.

The type of fast that you follow is going to determine what you can have and still maintain for the fast. For example, the regular alternate day fast would have you eat nothing on your fasting days, but the modified version allows you to have up to 500 calories during those fasting days.

On all forms, though, when you are fasting and not eating the one meal allowed, you are required to abstain from food and any drinks that have extra sugars and calories. Let's take a closer look at what is allowed when you are fasting and how to make sure you maintain your fasted state.

The Fasted State

With most forms of an intermittent fast, you will be required to separate your eating and fasting periods. During the eating periods, you are allowed to eat the amount of whole and nutritious foods that the body needs to stay healthy. The more that you can fill up on wholesome foods, the better you will feel when you get to your fasting window again. Focus on whole grains, lean protein, lots of fruits and vegetables, and some healthy dairy products if you can have them. Limit junk and processed food as much as possible.

When you are fasting, though, you need to maintain the fast. You should not eat anything during the fasting portion of this eating program. This allows the body to get into the fat burning state that it needs and can help you to cut down on calories. You can drink as much coffee, tea, and water as you would like to ensure that you stay hydrated.

When it comes to fasting, everything except the liquids that we mentioned before should be avoided. If special circumstances affect you, then you can take that into consideration and make some changes to your fast. But this is an exception and not the rule. For most people who go on an intermittent fast, it is best just to avoid eating anything and only consume the beverages that are listed above to ensure you don't enter dehydration.

If you can put something in your mouth, then it is often going to be considered as something that you should have while you are on your fast. This can include any food and snacks as well as breath mints, gum, and so on. Some fasting protocols may allow for you to consume these products and not consider it as breaking your fast. However, for the most part, it is best to abstain from anything except the non-caloric beverages. Exceptions can be made to things like medication. If you need to take a certain medication each day, you may want to consider following the 5:2 diet or modified alternate fast so that you can take some food in along with your medication to avoid making yourself sick in the process. Supplements and other similar products should be avoided as well until you can eat something with them.

The idea of bulletproof coffee has been introduced recently, and many people wonder if it should be counted as something that breaks the fast. It is coffee, which is one of the beverages allowed during your fast, but this kind of coffee adds in other ingredients that add to your calorie count.

In most instances, you would count it as something that breaks your fast because it does contain other food items and calories as well. You could easily introduce it with the first meal you consume during the day and get the same results. However, if your protocol says that it is not breaking the fast, then it is fine to follow that rule of thumb as well.

The 5:2 Diet and Modified Alternate Fasting

With the modified alternate day fast and the 5:2 diet, there are slightly different rules. These methods do allow you to eat a little bit on your fasting day, but you must keep this to a minimum. You are not allowed to graze on them, and you can't just eat whatever you want, or you will end up back to your original state.

On both versions of intermittent fasting, you can consume up to 500 calories each day. With the 5:2 diet, most people will choose to go with two meals during the day that are 250 calories each. With the modified alternate fasting diet, it is recommended that you eat just one meal, preferably towards the end of the fast or before going to bed, that totals 500 calories. Both can be effective, so you can choose the method that works for you.

When you do eat on both modified versions, you need to make sure that your meals are as nutritious as possible. You will quickly find that eating a bunch of junk is not going to fill you up and can make your fast even more miserable when cravings begin. Think about it. Two donuts equal 500 calories; however, they are definitely not as filling and nutritious as some turkey or chicken, half a cup of fruit, half a cup of vegetables, and a glass of milk or another similar meal. Choose your meals wisely, and you won't feel as deprived when you are on the fast.

Outside of the 500 calories that you can consume on these modified versions, you need to stick with the same rules as the other fats. You are not allowed to eat anything during the fast. Supplements are often discouraged and should be saved for your eating window to avoid upsetting the stomach. Sodas and other sugary beverages should be avoided, but having water, tea, and coffee is just fine. If you have medications that you must take at certain times, then those are fine, but if you have some freedom in when to take them, wait until your eating window begins again.

Chapter 8 Can Intermittent Fasting Be Dangerous

Although most people can follow the intermittent fasting diet with minimal side effects and virtually no lasting side effects, some people might find themselves experiencing some. The most likely dangers that you could experience includes:

You Might Struggle to Maintain Blood Sugar Levels

Although the intermittent fasting diet tends to improve blood sugar levels in most people, this is not always true for everyone. Some people who are eating following the intermittent fasting diet may find that their ability to maintain a healthy blood sugar level is compromised.

The reason for why this happens varies. For some people, not eating frequently enough may encourage this to happen. For others, transitioning too quickly or taking on too intense of a fasting cycle too soon, can shock the body which in turn causes a strange fluctuation in blood sugar levels.

You Might Experience Hormonal Imbalances

A certain degree of fasting, especially when you build up to it, can support you in having healthier hormone levels. However, for some people, intermittent fasting may lead to an unhealthy imbalance of hormones. This can result in a whole slew of different hormone-based symptoms, such as headaches, fatigue, and even menstrual problems in women.

Again, the reason for the hormonal imbalance varies. For some people, particularly those who are already at risk of experiencing hormonal imbalances, intermittent fasting can trigger these imbalances to take place. For others, it could go back to what they are consuming during the eating windows. Eating meals that are not rich in nutrients and vitamins can result in you not having enough nutrition to support your hormonal levels.

If you begin experiencing hormonal imbalances when you eat the intermittent fasting diet, it is essential that you stop and consult your doctor right away. Discovering where the shortcomings are and how you can correct them is vital. Having imbalanced hormones for too long can lead to diseases and illnesses that require constant life-long attention.

Headaches

A decrease in your blood sugar level and the release of stress hormones by your brain as a result of going without food are possible causes of headaches during the fasting window. Problems may also be a clear message from your body telling you that you are very low on water and getting dehydrated. This may happen if you are completely engrossed in your daily activities, and you forget to drink the required amount of water your body needs during fasting.

To handle headaches, ensure you stay well hydrated throughout your fasting window. Keep in mind that exceeding the required amount of water per day may also result in adverse effects. Reducing your stress level can also keep headaches away.

Some people find that the transitioning period includes many headaches. These headaches are often a result of you being hungry as your body adjusts to your new eating schedule. Typically, these headaches are dull and should be manageable. If it is not, you may be experiencing excessively low blood sugars. If your headache is too intense, refrain from fasting and eat. It is better to skip your fasting cycle and eat if you are experiencing negative side effects, than it is to attempt to stick it out and experience adverse or potentially dangerous side effects.

If you are experiencing chronic headaches, you may also be experiencing dehydration. Dehydration is common in most people, but it can be especially prevalent in those who are fasting. Typically, eating encourages us to drink, too. This is how we "wash it down." When you are not eating, you may also forget to drink water. Setting reminders to drink water and remember to get at least 3L a day can support you in overcoming headaches that may be caused by dehydration.

Cravings

During your fasting periods, you might find that you have higher levels of desires than usual. This often happens because you are telling yourself that you cannot have any food, so suddenly you start craving many different foods. This is because all you are thinking about is food. As you think about food, you will begin to think about the different types of food that you like and that you want. Then, the cravings start.

Early on, you may also find yourself craving more sweets or carbs because your body is searching for an energy hit through glucose. While you do not want to have excessive levels of sugar during your eating window, as this is bad for blood sugar, you can always have some. The ability to satisfy your cravings is one of the benefits of eating a diet that is not as restrictive as some other foods are.

From a psychological angle, cravings are intensified because of a feeling of being deprived of what you love to eat. For example, telling you to keep away from eating chocolate will somehow make you want to eat chocolate even more because you are unconsciously trying to overcome the feeling of being deprived. Stopping yourself from eating at the usual times you have conditioned your body to received food will naturally make you crave food more at those typical eating times.

To effectively handle your cravings, keep your mind off of food during the fasting window. Ensure that during your eating window, you indulge a bit with what your body craves. This will help to dampen the longing for that thing. Remember that you are not dieting, but fast, so you shouldn't worry unnecessarily over what you eat. Your focus should be on when you eat.

Low Energy

A feeling of lethargy is not uncommon during fasting, especially at the start. This is your body's natural reaction to switching its source of energy from glucose in your meals to fat stored in your body. So, expect to feel a little less energized in your first few weeks of starting with intermittent fasting.

To troubleshoot the feeling of lethargy, try as much as possible to stay away from overly strenuous activities. Keep things low key. Spending more time sleeping or just relaxing is another right way to ensure that your energy reserves are not depleted too quickly. The first few weeks are not the time to test your limits or push yourself.

Foul Mood

You may find yourself being on edge during fasting, even if you are someone who is naturally predisposed to being good-natured. The reason for the feeling of edginess is straightforward. You are hungry, yet you won't eat, and you are struggling to keep your cravings in check, plus, you may already be feeling tired and sluggish. Add all of these to the internal hormone changes due to the sharp decline in your blood sugar levels, and it's no wonder why you may be in such a foul mood. Tempers can easily flare up, and you may be quick to become irritated. This is normal when beginning a fasting lifestyle.

To effectively troubleshoot this, do all you can to keep away from irritable people and situations. If you consider someone annoying, do your best to stay out of their company or else they are more than likely to set you on edge. Find a way to deliberately focus your attention on things that easily trigger a feeling of happiness in you. Consciously seeking ways to be appreciative of the things around you, as well as to being grateful about the simple things of life, will go a long way toward keeping you from being easily irritated.

To handle this cold feeling, you can put on extra warm clothing, stay in friendly places, or drink a hot cup of unsweetened coffee. Taking a hot shower can also reduce the coldness.

Excess Urination

Fasting tends to make you visit the bathroom more frequently than usual. This is an expected side effect since you are drinking more water and other liquids than before. Avoiding water to reduce the number of times you use the bathroom is not a good idea at all, no matter how you look at it. Cutting down water intake while you are fasting will make your body become dehydrated very quickly. If that happens, losing weight will be the least of your problems. Whatever you do, do not avoid drinking water when you are fasting. Doing that is paving the way for a humongous health disaster waiting to happen. You don't want to do that.

The best way to handle excess urination is to stay close to a bathroom or a toilet wherever you find yourself throughout the day. You should urinate when the need arises. There is no other healthy shortcut to it.

People who are intermittently fasting tend to drink a lot of water in between eating windows. That is if they remember to. Often, water is used as a way to fill up your stomach to avoid feeling hungry throughout the day. It can also support you in overcoming heartburn. As a result, water is a popular option for people who are intermittently fasting.

At first, you may even find yourself going as often as twice an hour! There truly is no way around this, as water is essential and you do not want to decrease your intake. This will likely be a symptom that you experience on an ongoing basis, but you should see it as a good sign. This proves that you are well-hydrated and taking good care of your body.

Heartburn, Bloating, and Constipation

Your stomach is responsible for producing stomach acid, which is used to break down food and trigger the digestion process. When you eat frequent meals, unusually large meals, regularly, your body is used to producing high amounts of stomach acid to break down your food. As you transition to a fasting diet, your stomach has to get used to not producing as much stomach acid.

You might also notice an increase in constipation and bloating. People who eat regularly consume high amounts of fiber and proteins that support a healthy digestion process. When you switch to the intermittent fasting cycle, you can still eat a high volume of fiber and protein. However, early on, you might find that you forget to. As you discover the right eating habits that work for you, it may take some time for you to get used to finding ways to work in enough fiber and protein to keep your digestion flowing.

Heartburn may not be a widespread adverse effect, but it does sometimes occur in some individuals. Your stomach produces highly concentrated acids to help break down the foods you consume. But when you are fasting, there is no food in your stomach to be broken down, even though acids have already been produced for that purpose. This may lead to heartburn.

Bloating and constipation usually go hand in hand and can be very discomforting to individuals who suffer from it due to fasting.

Heeding the advice to drink adequate amounts of water usually keeps bloating and constipation in check. Heartburn typically resolves itself quickly, but you can take an antacid tablet or two if it persists. You may also consider eating fewer spicy foods when you break your fast.

You Might Experience Low Energy and Irritability

Until now, your body has been used to having a constant stream of energy pouring in all day long. From the time you wake up until the time you go to bed, it has been receiving some form of power from the foods that you eat. So, when you stop eating regularly, your body grows confused. It has to learn to create its energy rather than rely on the heat being offered to it by the food that you are eating.

Depending on how you are eating, your body may also be growing used to consuming fat as a fuel source rather than carbohydrates. This means that, in addition to losing its primary energy source, it also has to switch how it consumes energy and where it comes from. This can lead to lowered energy for a while. Do things that exert the least amount of energy. If you are someone who regularly exercises and works out, reducing the amount that you work out or switching to a more relaxed workout like yoga can help you during the transition period.

You Might Start Feeling Cold

As you begin to adjust to your intermittent fasting diet, you might find that your fingers and toes get quite cold. This happens because blood flow towards your fat stores is increasing, so blood flow to your extremities reduces slightly. This supports your body in moving fat to your muscles so that it can be burned as a fuel to keep your energy levels up.

Lowered blood sugars from fasting can also lead to cold extremities. More so, it makes them feel more sensitive to the cold. Staying warm with tea, hot showers, and extra layers can help overcome this coldness. If you notice that it is particularly prominent or that it spreads beyond your fingers and toes, you might want to adjust your diet to ensure that you are not experiencing chronic low blood sugars. This will ensure that you continue effectively managing your symptoms without experiencing adverse or dangerous side effects from intermittent fasting.

You Might Find Yourself Overeating

The chances for overeating during the break of the fast are high, especially for beginners. Understandably, you will feel starving after going without food for longer than you are used to. It is this hunger that causes some people to eat hurriedly and surpass their standard meal size and average caloric intake. For others, overeating may be as a result of uncontrollable appetite. Hunger may push some people to prepare too much food for breaking their fast, and if they don't have a grip on their desire, they will continue to eat even when they are satiated. Overeating or binging when you break your fast will make it difficult to reach your goal of optimal health and fitness.

An excellent way to tackle this is by making adequate plans ahead of time and sticking to those plans. Plan the quantity of food to be prepared well ahead of the eating window. Take into consideration the type of food as well as the meal size to be eaten. Although it may not be feasible to continually eat only fatty foods, increasing the frequency as well as the number of healthy fats in your diet will help you to feel satiated quickly.

During the windows where you can eat, you might find yourself eating as much as you possibly can. This is often a natural response to the feelings of hunger that you have experienced during your fasting cycle.

Choosing healthier options and eating mindfully is a good way to overcome overeating habits. This can support you in selecting options that are going to nourish and help your body, as well as prevent overeating. When you eat slowly and mindfully, you can recognize when you are no longer hungry. As a result, you can set down the fork and stop eating. Eating healthier options and eating slowly are the best ways to avoid overeating so that you do not waste your fasting benefits on an excessively unhealthy diet during your eating windows.

Hunger Pangs

People who start intermittent fasting may initially feel quite hungry. This is especially common if you are the type of person who tends to eat regular meals daily.

If you start feeling hungry, you can choose to wait it out if you have an eating window right around the corner. However, if there is a more extended waiting period or you are feeling excessively hungry, you should eat. Feeling hungry to the point that it becomes uncomfortable or distracting is not helpful and will not support you in successfully taking on the intermittent fasting diet. This is a pronounced side effect of going without food for longer than you are accustomed to.

For many people, their bodies have been conditioned to eat at certain regular intervals. So, at those intervals, their hunger hormones kick into action and stimulate a feeling of hunger. They either respond by eating a full meal or grabbing a quick snack. It is almost impossible not to feel very hungry when you attempt to break this pattern. Introducing fasting into your lifestyle is going to make you hungry. There are no two ways about it, and I'm not going to lie to you. The intensity of hunger is even higher when you are just starting. Hunger tests your resolve and mental toughness, especially in your first few days. This is the point where many will give up and walk away from their dreams and aspirations. But if you stay true to your resolve, hunger has a way of waning over time.

To reduce the hunger pangs, keep yourself occupied in some way throughout your fasting window. Keeping yourself busy, in addition to drinking water whenever you feel bouts of hunger, will help to keep your mind off food as well as suppress the appetite. Another way to troubleshoot hunger is to make sure you eat enough healthy fats, proteins, and fiber the day before you begins fasting.

The method of fasting that you opt for is entirely up to you. Hunger pangs are quite familiar during the initial week of fasting; don't get scared. Your body isn't used to starvation, and it will take a while to condition yourself to the diet. A hunger pang doesn't always indicate hunger. Confusing isn't it? At times, you will feel hungry when you are stressed or even bored. It is essential that you realize the difference between actual hunger and a natural craving. Ignore these pangs and get on with your day. Intermittent fasting doesn't mean that you should starve yourself, but at the same time, you shouldn't indulge in mindless eating either.

Chapter 9 How Intermittent Fasting Affects Both Males And Females

It's common knowledge that hormones and genetics play different roles in both males and females. And when it comes to dieting, there usually tends to be some changes too. While some of them turn out to be more assumptions than reality, a few of them have certain amounts of truths to them.

The Female Hormones and IF

When it comes to hormones, women are more sensitive to the changes in the environment or diet. In cases where the body senses that it's underfed, it triggers the hunger hormones – leptin and ghrelin into acting accordingly.

When you consider why the female body acts differently from that of the male, you'll find out that it all stems from evolution. From an evolutionary viewpoint, the body always keeps the woman in prime baby-making condition to avoid reducing fertility during a period of stress or starvation. None of which are safe or ideal for a baby.

You might be wondering what exactly triggers the hormonal responses; I'll tell you.

- Certain kinds of illnesses like infection and inflammation
- Poor food choices or eating very little food
- Not getting enough sleep/rest
- Excessive amounts of exercise
- A high amount of stress from either exercising too much or from the mental state

Funny enough, most of the scientific evidence on why women shouldn't fast (or do it differently) is based on the studies carried out on female rats. Granted, most of the studies carried out on rats tend to be accurate, but in some cases, there might be some irregularities.

For one, during the study, the rodents only ate every other day for twelve weeks. And two weeks into the research, their hormones had already gotten off balance, which resulted in the ceasing of their menstrual period and shrinking of ovaries.

Rats only live for a few years, unlike humans, and a whole day of fasting for them is the equivalent of depriving an individual of food for a few days. When that happens, the body goes into starvation mode, throwing the bodily functions off-kilter. And it's certainly not recommended for women or men.

It is also good to point out that calorie restriction during intermittent fasting for humans isn't as drastic as what the rats are put through.

As a result of the differences between males and females, most articles suggest that women do the crescendo method instead of intermittent fasting. The crescendo style is kind of similar to the 16/8, 5:2, and alternate-day method, in that you fast for 12 to 16 hours non-consecutively. The theory behind this practice is that spacing out your fasting days would help you avoid shocking your hormones, or ramping up your appetite. Other variations of intermittent fasting techniques include the 14/10; where you fast for 14 hours and feed during the remaining ten.

Suggested Intermitted Fasting Methods for Women

Based on the research that states females need to take a more relaxed approach to fasting than men, here are some of the suggested practices to follow;

- The Crescendo Method

This involves abstaining from food for 12 – 16 hours for 2 – 3 days in a week. The whole idea here is to space the fasting days evenly and avoid doing it back to back. A typical example would be fasting on Monday,

Wednesday, and Friday, while eating normally on Tuesday, Thursday, Saturday, and Sunday.

- The 24-Hour Protocol

This method also known as the eat-stop-eat has to do with fasting for a full day once or twice in a week. A maximum of two times a week is suggested for females. It's usually advisable to start with the 14-16 hours fasts first and building up momentum gradually.

- The Modified Alternate-Day

In this version, you get to fast every other day but eat normally on the non-fasting ones. You're permitted to consume around 20-25% of your regular calorie intake during fasting days.

- Leangains Method (16/8)

It involves abstaining from food within a 16-hour window and then eating within the remaining 8 hours allocated for feeding. Individuals who haven't fasted before are recommended to start with the 14-hour fasts first before progressing.

- The Fast Diet (5:2)

Here you fast for two days and eat normally during the remaining five. Calories should be restricted to around 25% of your usual intake (between 500 – 600 calories).

It's advised that you allow one day between the appointed fasting days.

Intermittent Fasting and how it affects the Testosterone

A lot of male bodybuilders follow this fasting method for its effects on testosterone levels; seeing as it's crucial for growth and repair. While women have little amounts of the hormone, men have greater amounts of it since it fuels most of their development from puberty.

Testosterone supports and increases muscle mass and strength in males through the improved synthesis of protein. It blocks the uptake and storage of fat, burning it instead by increasing beta-adrenergic (fat-burning) receptors in the cells.

Aside from the obvious role of the hormone regarding blood flow and erections, it's also essential for the healthy production of red blood cells and good heart health. It also has positive effects on mental health and cognition, proper kidney function, and bone growth and density.

Fasting for twenty-four hours elevates the growth hormone (GH) levels up to 2000%. Testosterone and GH are entwined, supporting each other in penile function, muscle building, and improved cognition. It also increases the levels of luteinizing hormone (LH) by around 67%. LH is a T-precursor.

Fasting intermittently also regulates leptin levels, which then stimulate the secretion of testosterone from the hypothalamus. And since fasting burns body fat, and the less amount you have, the more testosterone you produce; which makes fasting highly recommended for men.

After all, is said and done, the fact still remains that everyone's system differs from the next person. What works for you might not work for another individual – male or female.

When you want to try out intermittent fasting, first pick a method that works for your lifestyle and body; something you're also comfortable doing regularly. If you're the kind of person that loves eating breakfast, you could still use the 16/8 method and skip dinner instead. And if you feel the 14/10 practice works better for you, feel free to go for it. But always remember never to overdo anything.

Chapter 10 What Makes Intermittent Fasting the Best Way To Lose Weight

This is the question most people ask before jumping into the intermittent fasting bandwagon. The reason is simple. There has been a lot of buzz around intermittent fasting that it can become difficult to tell it apart from other weight loss diet fads. Intermittent fasting isn't a product; rather, it involves a lifestyle change that requires you to review the times you eat so that you're alternating between periods of fasting and eating. Generally, you'll have more hours of fasting compared to your hours of eating. As a result, you'll experience fat loss because your body is burning and using the stored fat for its fuel when you're in the fasted state. You don't have to make any drastic changes to your lifestyle like the foods you eat or even take chemicals or supplements to speed up the manifestation of the benefits.

Unlike many diet fads you may have tried before, intermittent fasting continues to deliver results for many people. The secret to succeeding with this method of health and wellness is to begin gradually, listen to your body, and make adjustments where necessary. Interestingly, intermittent fasting isn't based on restricting calories. It also doesn't dictate the kind of food you should eat. Instead, you eat your foods normally, so you don't have to give up some foods. Calorie restriction takes place naturally since you have a shorter feeding window. This pattern of feeding helps you to live a healthy lifestyle. This is unlike most diets that leave you with the temptation to eat more than you did before hence resulting in weight gain. Intermittent fasting is easy to follow through because all you need to do is pay attention to when you eat. Moreover, you're free to take fluids during your fasting window, so that eliminate the possibility of binge eating during the feasting window. There are various disadvantages of eating continually, particularly those foods containing free radicals. Thus, taking a rest from eating allows your body to rest from digestive processes. If you're not sure about embracing intermittent fasting for weight loss, here are some reasons you should consider this pattern of eating over dieting:

It's convenient. Diets can be demanding. In fact, one of the main reasons why most people abandon diets is because of the inability to follow through. Meeting various life's daily demands that require your attention alongside dieting can be a huge challenge. Intermittent fasting frees up the time you'd have spent preparing meals because you're essentially skipping a number of meals in a day. This means you have fewer instances of decision making. Moreover, you don't have to worry about moving away from your usual food choices as long as you're emphasizing on eating healthy whole foods. This is contrary to most diets that happen to be complex and expensive altogether, yet they don't produce the desired results.

Fasting strengthens your will power. Your intermittent fasting success is dependent on self-discipline. Intermittent fasting calls for you to be able to resist food even when you're tempted to eat. In the long run, this strengthens your capacity to stay focused and ignore distractions not just with food but other areas of your life as well. This eventually improves your ability to stay focused and focus on achieving your goals. When you fast, you become more alert and focused; thus, you can ignore any distractions that may come your way to achieve a set goal.

It's a great way to transition into a healthy lifestyle. Let's face it, most people find it difficult to stick to eating unprocessed foods even though they desire to. After all, processed foods are easily accessible, and they taste better. Intermittent fasting is a great way towards a lifestyle change because while it doesn't explicitly spell out the foods you should eat or avoid, you'll have better results when you include healthy foods in your meals. When your body adjusts to a shorter feeding window, you eliminate the temptation of eating junk food when hunger strikes.

It saves you money and time. Diets are generally expensive because you have to shop for specific food items and follow the menu to the latter in order to get certain results. This is in addition to the time you'll spend in meal preparation throughout the day. This is usually draining and a burden to your lifestyle. By fasting, you get to save resources and time.

A structured way of eating. When you're on a normal eating regimen, you're likely to keep on snacking mindlessly. In fact, you'll be surprised to learn that there's always something you can nibble on. Eventually, you end up putting on weight. Fasting helps you to have a structured pattern of eating.

Bigger meals are more satiating. Unlike the regular eating regimen where you're constantly thinking about food, intermittent fasting lets you have bigger meals which are more satiating because you'll be fuller for longer.

You can incorporate it into your social gatherings. When you're on a diet, it's unlikely that you'll be able to fit into social gatherings without having to worry about what you'll eat. With intermittent fasting, you can work out your schedule in a way that your feeding window falls within the time when you're most likely to attend social gathers. This way, you won't have to miss out on special occasions or even go out with friends.

You can fast and travel the world. If you love to globe-trot, you don't have to worry about putting off your intermittent fasting plan. Actually, intermittent fasting offers you a lot of flexibility that allows you to fast wherever you are. This means that you can maintain your lifestyle while at the same time, be able to enjoy new experiences and cuisines. Most importantly, you don't have to give up on this new way of life because you're traveling.

Heightened hunger awareness. Feelings of thirst and hunger are processed by the same part of your brain. As such, it's common to find that you're eating after every two hours because of other reasons that are manifesting as hunger. This could be feelings of boredom, stress, sadness, or happiness. Did you know that the smell of food can make you assume you're hungry? When you fast, your hunger awareness is heightened so that you actually know what it feels like to be hungry and can differentiate between the feel of hunger that is linked to other factors.

Improved quality of sleep. Most people who adopt the intermittent fasting lifestyle are motivated by the desire to shed excess weight. This might also be a case for you. What you don't know is that with it comes other benefits like better sleep. The reason for this is simple. When you're fasting, your body will mostly digest food before you go to bed. When your fat and insulin levels are kept in check, the quality of your sleep improves.

What Intermittent Fasting Does to your Body

Imagine having to wait for 16-18 hours before having your next meal. Well, that pretty much puts intermittent fasting into perspective - time-restricted eating. Understanding the science behind intermittent fasting is the first step towards reaping the benefits it promises. When you eat, your body releases insulin that is instrumental in the conversion of sugars into energy. The glucose that is not used is stored as fat. When you fast, you're naturally restricting calories; therefore, insulin is not released. What this means is that you can't lose weight unless your insulin levels go down. This explains why eating small meals all through the day isn't helpful when it comes to weight loss. When your insulin levels go down, it causes your body to respond by tapping into the fat stores in the liver and muscles for energy. When it exhausts these sources, it enters a state known as ketosis. This is where the liver breaks down fat to produce ketones that are used as a source of energy. Moreover, ketones are also known for their role in lowering appetite, reducing oxidative stress and inflammation levels. Ketones are also a source of a number of other benefits like a reduction in the risk factors for conditions like type 2 diabetes and heart disease.

Benefits of Intermittent Fasting

Intermittent fasting continues to take the health and fitness world by storm ostensibly because of its benefits. Most people who have tried losing weight over the years are often drawn to intermittent fasting because of the benefits it offers then go beyond losing weight. These benefits include the following:

Accelerated weight and fat loss. A 2017 study that was published in the journal of research found that intermittent fasting will help you lose weight even without having to count calories. This is based on the fact that during intermittent fasting, you have a shorter window within which you can eat your meals and achieve your daily calorie consumption. Eventually, this will reduce your calorie consumption naturally because it's utterly impossible to squeeze 4000 calories in your meals within a 4-hour window. This means that you will have a calorie deficit leading to significant loss of weight. In scientific terms, when you reduce your consumption of food, your blood insulin decreases paving the way for the process of breaking down fat for glucose to give energy. Eventually, your levels of cholesterol and triglycerides decreases. Even then, you must recognize that intermittent fasting is not a magic bullet for obesity and weight loss. Rather, it's a realistic approach that you can consider.

Improved cardiovascular health. Heart disease is a leading killer disease in the world. A study investigating the health benefits of intermittent fasting among non-obese individuals found a significant reduction in the level of triglyceride in men. On the other hand, women experienced an increase in good HDL cholesterol. This change was attributed to a 4% decline in body fat. Intermittent fasting ameliorates risk factors linked to a number of heart diseases by inducing stress resistance that has a cardioprotective effect.

Increased longevity. It may sound ironical that abstaining from food can actually increase longevity. Fasting has proven to increases the lifespan of various organisms like yeast and worms, among others. While intermittent fasting doesn't explicitly focus on calorie reduction, it shortens the feeding window, which eventually has an effect on the number of calories you can consume in a day. As a result, you get to enjoy better insulin sensitivity and a decline in the free radical damage to proteins and DNA, the body's cellular components. The result of this is lowered heart rate and blood pressure as well as a decline in incidences of spontaneous and induced tumors. Your body also becomes more resistant to neurodegenerative diseases. When you're in the fasted state, your body responds by producing various chemicals as a protective measure. These chemicals shield you from the side effects of fasting in addition to helping you fight depression and anxiety. They also help the body to become resistant to stress, thus slowing down the aging process; thus, promoting longevity.

Improved brainpower. Intermittent fasting boosts neuronal usefulness that frequently diminishes with the progression of age. As you advance in age, your dendritic spines begin diminishing. This influences the productivity of neural procedures significantly. Intermittent fasting will counteract the decrease of the dendritic spines density. A study of rats that were on an ordinary eating regimen revealed a 38% decrease in the number of dendritic spines. On the other hand, the rats that were on intermittent fasting had a close insignificant distinction in a youthful rodent that following 24 hours. It's worth noting that the rats also had improved learning capacities. The decrease in calorie consumption that is activated by intermittent fasting expands the procedure of neurogenesis, which is basically the arrangement of new brain cells, while likewise shielding the neurons from death. Moreover, it invigorates the generation of Brain-Derived Neurotropic Factor (BDNF), a protein that is connected to the expansion during neurogenesis. This hinders the neuron degenerations and aging. The impact on neurogenesis supports functional recuperation just as the mending of any harm to the spinal cord, notwithstanding whether intermittent fasting is introduced before or after injury.

Decreased persistent illnesses. Obesity and painful arthritic conditions are inflammatory diseases that are common today. Intermittent fasting reduces unnecessary inflammation and the risk of developing diseases associated with it. This means that intermittent fasting is able to improve long term health. A number of intermittent fasting methods have been tested to determine their effectiveness in disease control, and the results have been the same.

Better immune and inflammatory responses. The immune system is complex, yet it's what keeps the body from yielding to the onslaught of pathogens around you daily. However, it also could turn against the body and launch an attack at any time. Inflammation refers to the gathering of the white blood cells as well as other immune responses to eliminate and attack any threats to the body. A 2012 study on 50 people who observed Ramadhan, to analyze how their bodies responded to fasting, revealed that there was less inflammation during fasting. This study also noted diastolic and systolic blood pressure, the percentage of body fat and body weight reduced significantly. This decline was only notable when the participants fasted as the markers were higher again when they ceased fasting.

Chapter 11 Intermittent Fasting for The Overworked & Stressed-Out Woman

At this point, you surely have a solid foundation of knowledge about intermittent fasting under your belt, and you likely have decided on whether or not you'll attempt IF yourself. If you decided that IF is right for you, the method that's best for you has probably been settled upon at this juncture. Now comes the serious part.

There are times in a woman's life when intermittent fasting creates certain issues that need to be addressed with alterations to the fast, its length, or its strictness. For women who lead very stressed-out or overworked lives, intermittent fasting can be both helpful and hurtful but only if not practiced in the correct, most health-oriented ways. This chapter is dedicated to hashing out intermittent fasting's effects on everyday and long-term stress. It will explore how you can add IF to your life alongside daily stress without making things worse, and it will provide details on what foods and IF methods are best-suited for healing in your case.

By the end of this chapter, you should be confident that you can move forward with intermittent fasting despite stresses in your life. If you have anxiety, if you have a demanding work life, if you are often stressed-out, intermittent fasting can still be right for you! In fact, IF can even help people who lead high-stress lifestyles. It all depends on the approach.

IF & Its Effects on Stress

It is true that intermittent fasting poses a certain "stress" to the individual's system, but it does so in the same way that exercise works on the body. The trick for both is appropriate and health application and dosage.

Bodily "stress" as we feel it, regarding anxiety and frustrations, is triggered by the hormone cortisol, and intermittent fasting itself does not decrease that stress response in the body. What it does do is decrease the stress our cells experience as they age and deal with chronic disease. This type of stress is called oxidative stress, and it occurs when free radical molecules, which are unstable and problematic, interact with and do damage to the body's more important molecules, such as proteins and DNA.

A study conducted in 2005 on rodents and monkeys, and then another conducted in 2007 on human asthma patients, revealed that intermittent fasting might help make our cells more resistant to oxidative stress as well as inflammations within the body. The 2005 study additionally reveals how intermittent fasting even acts on the brain in ways that could decrease depression on the long-term for practitioners!

Essentially, these studies reveal how intermittent fasting makes the body oriented to work against aging and disease, to jolt itself back to life, and to remember how to heal itself. Given this effect in the body, it may be true that intermittent fasting doesn't help with overall stress, but it does work to heal things internally in a way that eases overall stress over time, depending on your situation, your personality, and how often you choose to fast.

How to Start Without Adding More Stress

If you experience intense stress periodically, daily, or chronically, you will have a unique relationship with intermittent fasting. I cannot lie, this practice of patterned timing with eating will add a degree of stress to your day. Following an extra routine, being sure to get the right calories, eating at the right times, etc., all these details will add to your tensions, but at the same time, the right application of the practice can be calming and affirming as you move forward. It can even be healing, as we learned with the 2005 rodent and monkey study.

The key is to remember that fasting is not the end-all, be-all answer to heal your stress. When applied to your life one or two weeks a month, IF can provide a healthy jolt to your cells and system overall. However, if you are a chronically stressed individual, when you start keep your demands on yourself with IF low (if you even choose to attempt it).

To incorporate IF into your routine without adding more stress, start by using day-by-day fasting methods instead of eating-window, daily methods. Once you settle into a day-by-day method that feels right, you can see what 16:8 or 14:10 feels like as long as your body approves.

Finally, for those who experience no restriction due to a relative lack of stress in their lives, you won't really have to worry about using a specific method to avoid excess stress. If you're looking for a high-energy routine that does stress you out, so to speak, then go ahead and choose in that respect.

Best Foods & Drinks to Incorporate

For people who experience a lot of stress whether periodically, daily, or chronically, it may be the case that now isn't the right time for you to try intermittent fasting. On the other hand, you might want to try it just a day or two a week and learn more about nutrition in the meantime. This section will be of great help to people in your situation, for it will provide some quick and easy facts about the foods and drinks you can incorporate to de-stress and emotionally or mentally de-clutter your life.

Asparagus is naturally high in folate, which helps one stay calm amongst stressors.

Avocado is high in glutathione, vitamins E & B, folate, beta-carotene, and lutein, all of which help you stay immune to stress.

Beans are a great source of magnesium, which helps with any body aches associated with working out or fasting as well as reverse the effects of stress by regulating blood pressure and cortisol, and they're also relatively high in tryptophan, which increases serotonin in the brain and enhances mood.

Berries are incredibly high in antioxidants as well as vitamin C, which lowers blood pressure and levels of cortisol, the body's stress hormone.

Brown Rice is a great source of magnesium, which helps with any body aches associated with working out or fasting as well as reverse the effects of stress by regulating blood pressure and cortisol.

Carrots are high in beta-carotene but crunching away at a raw carrot can also be relaxing, just like chewing on ice – only healthier and much better for your teeth.

Chocolate, dark chocolate, in particular, increases serotonin (which makes for better moods) and decreases cortisol (that pesky stress hormone); it can also help lower blood pressure due to the powerful antioxidants present in this tasty treat.

Fatty Fish like salmon is great for helping with stress because it's high in omega-3s, and it's also relatively high in tryptophan, which increases serotonin in the brain and enhances mood.

Garlic is high in antioxidants and helps to neutralize those free radicals that cause oxidative stress on our cells. Garlic heals both types of "stress"!

Grass-Fed Beef is a great source of vitamins C, B, E, and beta-carotene, and it's also packed with omega-3s while being relatively low in fat.

Leafy Greens are high in magnesium, which helps with any body aches associated with working out or fasting as well as reverse the effects of stress by regulating blood pressure and cortisol, and they're also filled with healthy fiber!

*Milk (*not as a drink during fast but with meals*)* is high in vitamins D & B and is a great source of protein to combat stress' effects in the body.

Nuts are high in omega-3s as well as potassium and zinc, which makes them a great immunity booster against stresses of all kinds. They are also relatively high in tryptophan, which increases serotonin in the brain and enhances mood.

Oatmeal is a great source of fiber and helps to boost energy through its grainy potential, and oats are also relatively high in tryptophan, which increases serotonin in the brain and enhances mood.

Oranges are high in vitamin C, which helps strengthen one's stress response.

Oysters are an incredible source of zinc, which boosts one's immunity, protecting against all sorts of future stress.

*Probiotics (*drink during fast & with meals; eat with meals too*)* are unparalleled in their abilities to mitigate anxiety and alleviate stress levels. They can even enhance one's mood.

Red Peppers are high in vitamin C, which helps strengthen one's stress response.

Seeds are a great source of in magnesium, which helps with any body aches associated with working out or fasting as well as reverse the effects of stress by regulating blood pressure and cortisol, and they're also relatively high in tryptophan, which increases serotonin in the brain and enhances mood.

Soy Beans, whether eaten as edamame, tofu, or miso, are relatively high in tryptophan, which increases serotonin in the brain and enhances mood. When fermented in miso, soybeans become probiotic, which makes them work to block stress all the better!

*Teas (*drink during fast & with meals)* of all kinds help the drinker de-stress through lowered cortisol in the body. Even caffeinated teas, such as black tea, were able to decrease the stress response for many drinkers. More commonly, however, decaf teas do the trick faster with less potential to fail. Try chamomile, green, peppermint, or ginger teas to soothe and heal from within against more than just stress.

Turkey is packed with tryptophan, which increases serotonin in the brain and enhances mood as well as makes you feel sleepy after eating so much of it on Thanksgiving or Christmas day.

Whole Wheat provides a great energy boost as well as demonstrates a perfect source of fiber to keep the body running in tip-top shape.

Yogurt, like milk, is high in vitamins B & D as well as protein to help combat the effects of stress on one's body. Most yogurts are also probiotic!

Best Fasting Method for You

For the generally unstressed woman, the crescendo method is a great place to start, but really, any method can work well for you to help decrease stress and increase overall healing. If you want an extra challenge, try 20:4. This method will certainly give you something to work for!

For the periodically stressed-out woman, try starting with the crescendo method, but if you like, you can alter your plans and try methods 5:2, alternate-day, or eat-stop-eat. These methods seem to have more balance between structure and flexibility, while crescendo requires a little more vigor than this individuals' other approved methods will.

For the daily stressed-out woman, the ideal method for intermittent fasting will be something that's fairly low-maintenance and low-stress to begin with. Through alternate-day, 5:2, and eat-stop-eat, these individuals should be able to use meal skipping to ease into day-by-day fasting (rather than eating-window, which can be more anxiety-inducing for these types of people).

Finally, for the chronically stressed-out woman, the ideal method, if you should choose to pursue intermittent fasting at all, will be one that hardly demands forethought. Spontaneous skip method is absolutely best-suited for this type of individual, but if that style of intermittent fasting seems to work well and the individual wants more of a challenge, he or she can easily switch to 5:2 method and practice it only one or two weeks a month to start.

Chapter 12 How to Set A Healthy Lifestyle with Intermittent Fasting?

In our world today, the standard of beauty and what constitutes the ideal physique has promoted and even praised unrealistic expectations for men and women alike. Everywhere you look there are cover models on magazines with chiseled abs, models fitting perfectly in size zero dresses, actors in every movie with physiques the average person could probably never obtain. Being exposed to this sort of standard from every angle day after day, can most definitely wear on our self-image and confidence.

Like I said, this goes for both men and women, but I think we can all agree that women bear the brunt of this aspect of life. The media does its very best to make you believe that you cannot be considered pretty, or in shape, unless you mimic these unrealistic expectations presented to you in the magazines and television. Sadly, this not only leads to lowered self-esteem in large numbers of women, but sometimes it can escalate into health disorders.

To try and cope with these expectations, some individuals develop a severe eating disorder known as bulimia. This is a disorder where someone consumes usually a large amount of food, feels guilty, and then becomes so worried that it will be detrimental to their physique that they actually induce vomiting, or take a large amount of laxatives, in a desperate attempt to reverse the situation. These methods are usually referred to as "purging." This disorder can wreak absolute havoc on the body. People with bulimia commonly have severe stomach distortion from overeating, electrolyte imbalance from severe dehydration, ulcers covering the lining of their esophagus from the constant stomach acid coming up from vomiting, and tooth decay also due to stomach acid. Although men and women both suffer from this disorder, women are much more prone to it. The United States Department of Health and Human Services reports that as many as 2% of women suffer from this eating disorder.

Another severe eating disorder many people suffer from is anorexia. This results in a person limiting their food intake to dangerously low levels for fear of gaining weight, exercising far too much in an attempt to burn calories. They often have a severely distorted body image in which they feel that their obese, when in reality they are far too thin. Once again, even though this disorder affects both men and women, it is predominately a female condition, with an estimated 1 in 20 women in the United States suffering from anorexia. This disorder also has terrible health implications such as heart problems, anemia, and extremely high-risk pregnancies.

Eating disorders are a real problem, and women are overwhelmingly more prone to developing them. So, how does all of this information relate to intermittent fasting, you may wonder? Well, my point is that with the way intermittent fasting places on emphasis on specific periods of fasting, followed by strict eating windows, it can sometimes cause women to develop an unhealthy obsession with food.

If your body is still getting used to going extended periods of time without eating, there is a greater likelihood that when the feeding window begins you will be so hungry that you overdo it. If you are really wanting to see results from following this protocol and are ashamed of yourself for consuming an excessive amount of food, the guilt you feel might even lead you to becoming bulimic, purging yourself to try and undo the situation. Likewise, if after adhering to intermittent fasting for some time and not seeing the results that you hoped for, you may start to feel like what you are doing is not enough. This can cause women to become more predisposed to developing anorexia.

When this happens, it is easy to see how someone may shorten their eating window far too much, or barely eat any food at all during the allotted feeding time. Although women must be aware and cautious of these eating disorders when beginning intermittent fasting, this becomes even more important if they have any prior history of eating disorders, as the likelihood of relapsing increases substantially. To prevent any of these eating disorders from rearing their ugly head, one needs to make sure that their perspective is in the right place. The first thing you need to remember is that intermittent fasting is about becoming a healthier, happier version of you.

Well these don't mean anything if you develop an extremely unhealthy relationship with food in the process. It is important that you keep in mind why you started it in the first place; to better yourself. The second thing to keep in mind is that you are a human being (shocker, right?). We are imperfect creatures with limited self-control, we make mistakes.

I can assure you that if you choose to begin intermittent fasting, there will be times that you make mistakes. Maybe that eating window just cannot wait, and you give in to the hot and ready sign at Krispy Kreme on your way home. Sometimes you may consume a few too many calories when those precious feeding hours begin. In nutrition, fitness, and even life in general, it is never the small, infrequent things that yield long term results. What you need to remember is that the things you do HABITUALLY are what will make or break you.

If you eat a terrible diet routinely and randomly decide to eat healthy for only one day, do you think you are going to immediately lose 10 pounds? Is going to the gym twice a year going to get you in fantastic shape and allow you to reach your fitness goals? Having said that, slipping up on your diet from time to time or missing a workout every once in a while, is not going to ruin your weight-loss and exercise goals. Anything worth achieving, especially when it comes to your body, is not going to happen overnight.

However, if you consistently follow the intermittent fasting protocol, or any other diet for that matter, then even with the minor setbacks that happen you are still on the path to your goals! When it comes to intermittent fasting, you need to understand that this is merely a tool at your disposal that you are choosing to use to become a healthier person. You must never let something like this control you, after all, you are the one in control choosing to live this lifestyle, and you have the power to stop or change the rules at any time.

In your journey with intermittent fasting, it is of the utmost importance that you never lose sight of the big picture. Remember that food is not the most important thing in your life, and preoccupation with eating should never get in the way of the things that matter most to you. Although cruel, societal definitions and images portrayed by the media are giving us a horrible definition of what it means to be healthy.

If you let it, comparing yourself to these people will do nothing but rob you of your joy and discourage you from trying to be your best. The only measuring stick that you should stand next to in your journey should be your former self. It is amazing how much fitness and nutrition mirror all of life itself. In everything you do, you should wake up every morning trying to improve yourself from the you that fell asleep last night. Never let anyone tell you that you are not good enough and that you're not capable of reaching your health and wellness goals. You are more than capable of achieving them with the right amount of knowledge and commitment.

Chapter 13 Intermittent Fasting And Ketogenic Diet Combined

Many people are not familiar with the ketogenic diet. A ketogenic diet is like every diet only it triggers ketone bodies made by the liver, move the body's metabolism to fat utilization from glucose use. It restricts carbohydrate intake to a low level that causes certain reactions. It is however not a high protein diet. It is a moderate-protein, low-carbohydrates, and high-fat diet. The exact macronutrient ratio will differ according to your needs as an individual. In a basic ketogenic diet, fat makes up seventy-five percent of the calories you take, proteins make up thirty percent of calories you take calories and carbohydrates make up ten percent of calories you take.

Normally the body functions on a mix of proteins, fats, and carbohydrates. This diet removes carbohydrates thus cause the body stores to get depleted making the body to find an alternative source of energy. It can use free fatty acids for most bodily organs but not all for example brain and nervous system, but they can use ketone bodies.

Incomplete free fatty acid breakdown releases ketone bodies as a by-product. The energy provides to organs like the brain as fat derived non-carbohydrates. Ketosis develops as a result of accelerated production of ketone bodies making them accumulate in the blood. There is also reduced glucose production and use in the body and reduced protein breakdown for energy.

Ketogenic diets affect insulin and glucagon levels. Insulin turns glucose to glycogen which is stored as fat while glucagon turns glycogen to glucose to provide energy for the body. Removal of carbohydrates in the diet increases glucagon levels but reduces insulin levels. This results in more free fatty acids being released and their burning in the liver thus leading to the manufacture of ketone bodies and induces the metabolic state ketosis.

In all diets, exercise will help in fat burning; the ketogenic diet is the same. However, sustaining high-intensity exercise can be challenging as the diet does greatly reduces carbohydrate intake, but low-intensity exercise is okay. There are various versions of the ketogenic diet there are others that allow carbohydrates.

There is no one-size-fits-all when it comes with how much of your total calorie requirement you should derive from carbohydrates. Some nutritionists' advice that people to keep it in the low end, which is five percent, but it is not necessarily good advice as the exact amount depends on your body. To get the right amount for you will have to rely on the trial and error method. Select a percentage and see how it feels for you if you do not like the results you can adjust accordingly. With fats and protein, just like in carbohydrates, there is no exact amount for everyone. It all depends on you, but seventy-five percent is a good place to start off.

Like in intermittent fasting, there are foods that you should eat and others you should avoid. In this diet, there are some foods which are on the fence between being allowed and not be allowed and there are others that are totally off-limits. The macronutrient ratios help you determine if a food is allowed or not.

Quality of food matters more than quantity here. The ideal foods include grass-fed and pasture-raised meat, eggs from pasture-raised hens, grass-fed butter and cheese, fruits, organic creams, and vegetables. They are ideal but even eating conventional foods will not stop ketosis from taking place. Do what you can to eat high-quality foods.

You should eat lots of fat in the ketogenic diet as they are the main source of energy, this does not mean that you can eat fat limitlessly. Some fats that are good for you and others are not. You are required to eat many saturated fats from poultry, eggs, meat, coconut and butter: polyunsaturated fats like tuna and salmon; and monounsaturated fats like nuts, nut butter, avocado, and olive oil. Highly processed polyunsaturated fats like vegetable oil and soybean oil should be avoided.

Protein can be obtained from many of the sources of fat like meat and eggs. You can also eat bacon and sausages for protein and fat. As your body turns excess protein to glucose, you should eat within the recommended grams of protein to keep you in ketosis.

Since fruits contain sugar, however natural they are they will increase your blood glucose and remove you from ketosis thus many of fruits are not recommended. Fruits are not totally banned; it depends on your intake. Fruits high in fiber and low in carbohydrates are best. Vegetables, on the other hand, are very important because they provide minerals and vitamins without adding many calories. They help you stay healthy. Some vegetables are full of carbohydrates so not all vegetables are allowed on the ketogenic diet. Eat leafy or dark green vegetables like spinach, broccoli, and green beans, asparagus, cucumbers, and mushrooms. Avoid starchy vegetables like white potatoes, yams, corn, and sweet potatoes.

In a ketogenic diet, full-fat dairy is regular. To assist you to meet your fat needs to use heavy cream, sour cream, hard cheese, butter, and cottage cheese. Avoid low fat and flavored dairy products, as they are full of sugar.

Water is the best beverage for you to drink. You should always strive to drink about half of your body weight in ounces. Unsweetened coffee and tea are allowed. Keep away from sodas, flavored water, sweetened lemon aid; fruit juices basically any sweet drink. To add excitement to plain water you can fuse it with fresh herbs.

Grains and sugars in all forms should be avoided. Grains are like rice, rye, wheat, sorghum, barley and any of their products. This translates to no pasta, bread, and crackers. Honey, brown and white sugar, corn syrup, maple syrup and anything else that contains sugar is not allowed. Make sure what you eat does not contain any form of sugar.

The bodily reactions caused by a ketogenic diet are closely like those that happen during intermittent fasting. The meager insulin feedback to dietary protein causing blood glucose to be cultivated at higher levels is the difference between ketogenic diet and fasting. The liver converting dietary protein to glucose causes this. At the same time, carbohydrate restriction decreases the insulin and cortisol simultaneously there is an increases growth hormone, glucagon, and adrenaline.

With the ketogenic diet, there is no room for 'cheating' your diet. You should strictly follow it since even one meal that does not follow its guidelines can slow your progress for about a week, as your body will have been removed from the ketosis state. Always ensure that you have eaten enough, and you are satisfied to prevent you from having a snack that could spoil everything you have been working for.

Intermittent fasting can aid you to reach ketosis faster that following a ketogenic diet on its own. This is possible as the body, when your practicing intermittent fasting, derives its energy from fats instead of carbohydrates. This is the same thing that the ketogenic diet strives to achieve. Therefore, it can help you if you find it challenging to get into a ketosis state.

Combining the two may result in faster fat burning than each on its own. Your body uses stubborn fat during intermittent fasting as it promotes metabolism resulting in heat production. This helps in preserving muscle mass during weight loss and improves your levels of energy benefiting keto dieters who desire to burn fat and better their athletic performance. Combining the intermittent fasting eating period system and ketogenic diet calorie counting and eating regimen can result in more body fat burning than people who still eat junk food.

It can also boost your physic as intermittent fasting increases the production of the human growth hormone but a very huge percentage. This hormone plays a huge role in muscle building. According to research done the human growth hormone makes a person have lower levels of body fat and increase lean body and bone mass. Working out in a fasted state can cause metabolic adaptations in your muscle cells resulting in fat burning for energy. The human growth hormone also helps you recover at a faster rate from injury or even hard work out. It also reduces skin inflammation and makes it supplier. It improves your skin's resistance to wrinkles and sagging.

The combination of the two can even have a positive effect on the aging process. They cause an increase in stem cell production. These are like building blocks to the body as they can be made into any cell that the body needs and replace old or damaged cells keeping you younger for longer internally. These stem cells can do wonders for your skin, old injuries, chronic pain, and many more. This can improve your life expectancy since your overall health is improved through blood glucose balance, reduced inflammation and better free radical defense.

It can stimulate autophagy. This is simple terms is cell clean up. When it begins, your cells move through your internal parts, remove any damaged or old cells, and put new ones in their place. It is like an upgrade for your organs. It reduces inflammation and increases the life of those organs.

When practicing the ketogenic diet and intermittent fasting, there are no cravings, fatigue and mood swings. This is achieved by constant low blood sugar levels. This is because fat does not increase your blood sugar levels. You will be able to maintain low blood sugar levels, which can greatly help with people with type 2 diabetes even, get off their medications.

The liver changes fat into energy bundles called ketones, which are released into the blood to give energy to your cells. These ketones suppress the main hunger hormone, ghrelin. High ghrelin levels make you hungry while ketones reduce the hormone levels even when there is no food in your digestive tract. This means that you can stay a longer period of times without eating and you will not get hungry. The ketogenic diet undoubtedly makes fasting much easier thus more manageable for you to do.

There are people who have incorporated intermittent fasting to the ketogenic diet. This is by following the dietary regulations of the ketogenic diet while also following the intermittent fasting eating pattern. This can have many benefits including high-fat burning rates since they both major on using fats for energy over carbohydrates, giving you energy, reduce cholesterol in the body, regulating your blood sugar which can help treat type 2 diabetes, will help deal with hunger, and reduce skin inflammation.

Combining the two is safe for most people and can greatly speed up the process of fat burning making you achieve your goal faster. It is, however, possible to do one or the other on their own as they have many similar benefits. It is also important to choose an intermittent fasting regiment that suits you and always make sure you eat enough of the macro foods. To put it to perspective, think of fasting as a bar of soap and ketogenic diet as a sponge. If you want to wash dishes, you can use the soap and sponge individually. Depending on what was in the dishes that can both do the work relatively okay. When you combine both, the work done will be perfect and will make cleaning a lot easier for you to do as they both work in different ways but complement each other superbly.

Chapter 14 Should I Add Any Exercise Into My Fast?

The most effective intermittent fast is one where you add lots of healthy exercises as well. Intermittent fasting can do a great deal of good when it comes to cutting calories and helping you lose weight, but the other part of the equation is for you to add in some exercise as well. Exercise can help you maintain your muscle mass, burn more calories than fasting alone and give you more energy to get through the day.

A common question that people on an intermittent fast may have is how they can add in more exercise to their day and which exercises are the best. To keep it simple, any exercise that you enjoy doing and that you will keep doing for the long term is going to be perfect. However, there are times when a specific workout will be more effective or enjoyable to you.

If you can, it is best to do a good mixture of workouts with some weight training, cardio, and strength training mixed together. But doing one type of exercise that you love is better than not doing anything at all. Let's explore some of the different types of workouts that you can consider with intermittent fasting, and how to do them safely to get the best results.

Weight Lifting and Intermittent Fasting

When it comes to intermittent fasting, many people like to begin a weight lifting or strength training workout. This can be beneficial in several ways. First, it helps you to build up lots of lean and strong muscles that make you look trimmer and can burn through more fat and calories than just intermittent fasting alone. Strength training can also work when you are in a fasted state because you don't need to burn up fuel as quickly as you do with cardio.

Many people who add weight training to their routine will do it while they are in their fasted state, although it is fine to add in anywhere you have time. Doing this during the fasted state can help you burn through even more glycogen than before, giving you better results.

If you do choose to weight train during a fast, try to set it up so that you end your fasting window right after the exercise is done. This way, you can get the benefits of training while fasted, but then you can provide the body with the nutrients it needs to repair those muscles once the workout is done.

With weight training and intermittent fasting, fewer reps with more weight are the best option. This helps you to get the stronger muscle that looks lean, without having to spend hours in the gym. Start out small, and perhaps even skip the workouts in the beginning. You will get stronger and will be able to take on more weight but remember that this is a time when your body is adjusting, and you never want to overdo it.

Is HIIT a Good Idea to Add into My Exercise Plan

One thing that you may want to consider adding into your exercise program is HIIT or high-intensity interval training. This type of exercise can really help add in many extra health benefits, and it doesn't require you spending hours in the gym like other methods.

Researchers have taken time to look at HIIT exercises and found that they can be effective. It has been shown that doing three rounds of 20 seconds of HIIT three times a week can give the body as many benefits as you get while running on the treadmill. Instead of spending all that time running on the treadmill or at the gym, you could spend about ten to 15 minutes on your workout and get the same benefits.

For those who are just getting started on their own intermittent fast and aren't used to the effects, or those who aren't used to doing a lot of working out, it can be great news to help them get started. You will get a ton of benefits with just a short burst of exercise, and who wouldn't want to see that?

You get some choices when it comes to HIIT. You can either make the whole workout based on this idea or find ways to add it into your regular workout. For example, you can either do ten minutes of the spurts or go out for a two-mile walk and add in three or four rounds with a sprint that lasts about 20 seconds each. Both will provide you with good benefits to your health in a shorter amount of time.

Do I Need to Worry About Preserving My Muscles During an Intermittent Fast?

Many experts agree that out of the health benefits that you get out of exercise and diet, 80 percent comes from your diet. The other 20 percent will come from the exercise that you do. This means that it is more important to concentrate on consuming the right kinds of foods to help you lose weight and keep your muscle strength intact. However, adding exercise to the mixture can really help you get healthier as well.

Some research looked at the data of participants who were on the show *The Biggest Loser*. The information that was looked at for this research included the resting metabolic rate, the total amount of energy used, and the total body fat of all the participants and these numbers were measured three times. They were measured right when the program began, after six weeks into the program, and then finally done after 30 weeks.

Researchers found that the diet the participants consumed was the most responsible for the weight that they lost. And only about 65 percent of that loss in weight came from body fat. The rest came from a loss in lean muscle mass. Exercise alone resulted in an only fat loss with a slight increase in lean muscle mass. This means that it is possible to lose a little bit of muscle mass with just diet alone but adding in exercise will ensure that you can maintain and even grow that muscle mass while eating a healthy diet like on an intermittent fast.

Chapter 15 Ifer's Vs. Low Carb Junkies

There are IFer's who will bash the low or no carb lifestyle and visa versa. And then there are those who somehow intertwine the two together.

Statesmen and women of both lifestyles can be seen all over the internet bashing one another giving claims that the others is not the healthiest choice to be making when it comes to long term health.

Those that utilize both will swear by the combination of intermittent fasting and carbohydrate reduction and its powerful effects on their inward and outward appearances.

Some medical and dietary science experts say that a person who is following a low carb or no carb diet for a prolonged period of time can start to develop an aversion for anything that is low carb.

They say that the people who completely avoid carbs for long periods of time will possibly experience a distaste for what they are consuming as their daily caloric intake which consists of fats and protein, and this can lead to drastic health issues. These experts believe that the body is meant to be fueled by carbohydrates.

Withholding carbohydrates from the body and depriving it of its natural fuel and energy source can start the domino effect of poor health and serious illnesses.

Back in 2003, the American Dietetic Association commented on low carb diets. They stated that, high carb foods have very limited effects on the body's fat storage mechanism since these are very good at enhancing insulin resistance.

Zero carb and low carb: According to the American Academy of Family Physicians, low carb diets include any diet that restricts carbohydrates and places them between 20 and 60 grams per 24 hour day. A no carb diet would be anywhere under 20 grams and many consider 30 – 40 grams to be a no carb diet.

It would be extremely difficult to get your carbs under 20 grams. There are also the no carb Atkins style dieters who will subtract the fiber grams off of their daily carb intake. So if they ate a total of 50 carbs and 30 of those grams were fiber, they would count their daily carb intake as 20 grams.

There is really no one size fits all low or no carb diet. Those considering this type of lifestyle should definitely get with their Doctors and get their advice.

Those that are intermittent fasting and also low or no carb dieting at the same time should definitely seek advice from their Physician and watch for any signs of fatigue, as this is a common complaint of those combining the two together, and this can lead to dangerous health problems down the road if the person continues this pattern.

Chapter 16 Ifer's Vs. Paleo Dieters

Just like with the low and no carb junkies, the paleo diet gets thrown into the mix when the term intermittent fasting is mentioned. And there are also people on both sides who bash one another, claiming that the other side is not the optimal choice for long term health.

And there are those who combine the two, and even those who combine all three together. There are people who follow the paleo diet, and low carb diet, and utilize IF patterns all simultaneously in conjunction with one another.

The *Paleolithic* diet also known as the *Cave Man* diet is often mistaken for another low or no carb diet. Although many people who follow this diet seem to tend to lean toward the low carb side, the paleo diet is in fact not a low carb diet.

In a nutshell the paleo diet is about bringing us back to our pre – historic ancestor times, when we were hunter gatherers. There are many variations of this diet as well.

Some people don't believe in eating anything that was not picked from a tree or caught on land. Others will eat things such as processed breads, beans, potatoes, and drink massive amounts of coffee and alcohol and call it paleo. There is a huge division in the paleo diet family as they are all trying to define paleo as their interpretation of the diet.

Many intermittent faster's seem to be attracted to this type of diet. Many have claimed of great results both in their physical appearance and mental status when combining the two together.

Many intermittent faster's praise the paleo diet for keeping them on what they call "clean" foods. Clean foods are basically another way of saying non – processed foods.

Even by following the most liberal of paleo diets you will avoid so many processed foods that contain additives, and preservatives, and refined sugars, and bad fats. These are some of the things that lead us down the road to poor health, and weight gain, and are the reason for many of people's illnesses.

Chapter 17 Ifer's Infatuation With Coffee & Stimulants

Like the paleo dieters intermittent faster's tend to be big caffeine and stimulant consumers. This may have to do with the fact that a lot of them will carb restrict as well.

The brain runs solely on glucose and oxygen. The human body was made to run on carbohydrates, this is a scientific fact. Restricting or completely eliminating carbohydrates from your diet just forces your body to turn stored fat into glucose for fuel.

If you eliminate fat as well then you will just be forcing the body to once again convert what is left which would be protein (muscle) into glucose, which is a more dangerous process then having your body convert fat into glucose. If you eliminate all three and don't consume any alcohol (calories) then the body will have to just die off.

There are people that may wonder how they can see drunken hobo's in their streets who basically live off of alcohol and maybe get a hot dog every now and then at the 7/11 still alive! Day after day, some even for years doing the same thing every day which is getting drunk out of their minds.

They will eventually die, but the alcohol they are consuming is also keeping them alive for the time being. Alcohol will turn into glucose in the body which is our primary and most needed source of fuel. Alcohol will also dehydrate you and disrupts and suppresses the body's natural process of protein synthesis. Myopathy is also a common condition found in alcoholics, but this is somewhat off subject and for another book and time.

Those who consume caffeine or other stimulants on a daily basis are wreaking havoc onto their adrenal glands. All across the world millions of people are waking up, rolling out of bed and the very first thing that they do is have a cup of coffee.

Many people have alarms set on their coffee makers so that their coffee starts and is finished brewing by the time that they are getting up for work or school or whatever their daily activity may be.

Intermittent faster's may find themselves in lethargic states of mind and feeling sluggish and weak if not practicing IF correctly. These people will need to turn to stimulants to get their brains kick started. Many people do not know the importance of the adrenal glands, and what role they actually play in our bodies.

Chapter 18 Misconceptions and Truths About Intermittent Fasting

In the health and wellness world, there is a lot of information to absorb, and some of it can be misleading. You are the expert on you, and it's up to you to decide what actions you will take in order to take care of your incredible body. Some of these well-meaning pieces of information contradict what you have learned about intermittent fasting so far—so to help you decide if intermittent fasting is for you, here are a few common misconceptions and how they relate to intermittent fasting.

You Can't Skip Breakfast

How many times have you heard, "Breakfast is the most important meal of the day?" That statement isn't wrong, but it's not entirely right, either. Every meal is the most important meal of the day—and whether you eat at 7am or 12pm, you are still having breakfast. The common belief is that skipping breakfast can lead to cravings and unbearable hunger—but with a few smart choices, such as a nourishing meal for dinner and using water to keep hunger at bay, waiting until later in the day to eat is not unbearable at all. It is a personal decision, and it is up to everyone to figure out the best time in their day to have breakfast.

Frequently Eating Will Boost Your Metabolism

Eating 3 meals a day and having small snacks in between has been a staple in the diet fad world for years, but it hasn't been proven to provide significant benefits to weight loss and can often lead to a feeling of overload and frustration. The theory was that frequent eating is what keeps the metabolism working and expending energy all day long, but this isn't true. The deciding factor in the body-mass composition is the total number of calories you consume—and if you consume more than you can use in a day, you will gain weight. There have been many studies done over the years, and there is no proof that increasing or decreasing the frequency of your meals has any effect on your metabolism. Through intermittent fasting, you generally eat fewer calories due to the time restraints— so the logic is weight loss is imminent, provided the calories you consume are healthy choices.

Eating Frequent Meals Is Better for Your Health

When the body has a constant stream of food to digest, it never gets a moment to perform important internal maintenance processes, such as cellular repair in a process called autophagy. This is where your cells seek out old and dysfunctional proteins and effectively remove them from your system so that they don't cause damage. It's the ultimate recycling program! Occasional fasting allows the body to redirect its focus from digestion to other vital processes that have a net benefit on your overall health. We have evolved from ancestors who hunted and gathered food and sometimes went long periods without a food source—and our bodies adapted to that. Only in our recent history have we had 24/7 access to nutrition, as well as the anti-nutrition of fast foods and processed meals. Give your body a break, and let it do what it was designed to.

Snacking Reduces Hunger

This is another topic that has mixed reviews—some studies suggest that frequent meals reduce hunger, while others suggest the opposite. This is again a highly personal issue and needs to be experimented with on a case-to-case basis and depends entirely on the foods snacked on. If you are choosing high-volume foods with fiber and protein, you will be fuller longer; if you snack on junk food, the hunger cravings will be immediate. Choose wisely, and don't worry about needing to fit 6 small meals into an 8-hour eating window.

Your Brain Needs a Constant Source of Glucose (a.k.a. Energy)

There is a theory that if the brain doesn't have a source of carbohydrates every few hours, it will stop functioning—this is based on the idea that the only energy source the brain can use is glucose (from carbohydrates), but the brain and your body are adaptable and can easily produce glucose from fat cells in a process called gluconeogenesis. This is the premise of the Keto diet, which limits carbs to a bare minimum to utilize this process to burn off excess fat. Keto and intermittent fasting can be used together to benefit from the combined effect of limiting carbs and managing blood sugar levels to achieve a body chemistry hack. This is considered a restrictive diet plan and should be approached cautiously and does not agree with everyone.

Fasting Is Starvation

One very common misconception is that through fasting your body will go into 'starvation mode' and will shut down your metabolism entirely—but studies have shown that short-term fasts increase your metabolic rate. When you fast, your metabolism turns to fat cells and breaks them down to access the energy stored within— this takes energy, so your metabolic rate must increase to perform the task. There is a fine line, though, and you can cross over into starvation mode if you fast for longer than 48 hours—at which point your metabolism will begin to decrease.

You Can Only Process a Certain Amount of Nutrients at a Time

Some experts claim that the body can only handle so much protein at a time, and trying to fit more in for every meal is just wasting it—but these are not experts, and there is no scientific evidence to support this claim. The number of macronutrients should be measured on a 24-hour timeline—and as long as you meet your target for daily nutrition, whether it is in a 12-hour window of just the 4-hour window in the warrior diet, your body will know what to do to maximize it all.

Fasting Leads to Overeating

This is a tricky one and not the answer everyone wants to hear—it is not the diet you are on that causes overeating. Rather, it is the choices you are making that leads to overeating. You can't blame a plan written on a piece of paper for the choice you make to eat a chocolate bar instead of an apple or that slice of pizza for breakfast instead of some nutritious avocado toast. Ultimately, your success is entirely up to you—and the more you practice self-discipline, the better you become at it. If you choose something that isn't aligned with your plan, do not beat yourself up about it—that choice is behind you, and you can always do better on the next one.

Conclusion

I hope this book helped you understand the basics of occasional fasting and the benefits that this diet will bring into your life. By practicing occasionally fasting while you are fit, without having to adhere to strict diets that can be harmful to your health, you will succeed in reducing weight and be in the best form of your life.

Understanding the principles of occasional fasting, will not only help to reduce your weight, but it will also contribute to the strengthening of your mental health by training your brain to be durable and to resist food in moments that are meant for fasting. This way you will become a stronger person. But the psyche is not the only thing that will be strengthened. Who does not want strong and well-shaped muscles? Well, occasional fasting will help in creating this. You must be wondering how can something that deprives you of food, helps you build muscle when you know that building muscle requires more calorie intake. Well, this is not the case. Basically, intermittent fasting will teach you to appreciate food and to refer to a healthy diet that will become part of your everyday life. With the right combination of fat, carbohydrates, protein, fresh fruits and vegetables, you will able to create meals that the body needs on the days of not fasting.

The next step is to list all the various methods of intermittent fasting once more, to help you choose the one that will best suit your lifestyle and daily responsibilities, and gradually start to change your life and take care of your health forever. Of course, do not be alarmed if you are suddenly unable to endure the whole fasting period. Allow your body some time to get used to this way of eating, and over time you will be able to lengthen the time for fasting. Combine some simple exercises to increase the burning of fat from your body, or prepare your own exercise plan that will fit your fitness level. But, try not to forget the recommendations given in the book of the combination of the intensity of exercise on the days when you are fasting and the days when you are not fasting.

It is important to plan exercise days wells. If you practice high-intensity workouts on the fasting day, you will feel exhausted, and your muscles will be under a lot of stress, which is not good when you are trying to shape and enhance. Also, to get those well established and toned muscles, drink plenty of water (at least eight glasses, but really this is the minimum amount we need) and remember to combine protein, carbohydrates, and fat before and after training to help your muscles grow. Take the recommendations for gradual entry into the process of fasting and become one step closer to changing your whole life and becoming happier and satisfied with your visual appearance and health.